# the hedonistic neuron

## a theory of memory, learning, and intelligence

**A. Harry Klopf**

Avionics Laboratory
Air Force Wright Aeronautical Laboratories
Wright–Patterson Air Force Base, Ohio

●HEMISPHERE PUBLISHING CORPORATION
A member of the Taylor & Francis Group

New York    Washington    Philadelphia    London

THE
HEDONISTIC
NEURON
A Theory of Memory,
Learning, and
Intelligence

 3 4 5 6 7 8 9 0   B R B R   8 9

This book was set in Press Roman by Hemisphere Publishing Corporation.
The editor was Christine R. Flint; the designer was Sharon Martin DePass;
the production supervisor was Miriam Gonzalez; and the typesetter was
Frederick Belmonte Wright.
Braun-Brumfield, Inc., was printer and binder.

**Library of Congress Cataloging in Publication Data**

Klopf, A. Harry, date.
  The hedonistic neuron.

  "A revised and updated version of Air Force Cam-
bridge Research Laboratories Special Report number 133
(AFCRL-72-0164), Brain function and adaptive systems—
a heterostatic theory."
  Bibliography: p.
  Includes Index.
  1. Brain. 2. Memory—Physiological aspects.
3. Learning—Physiological aspects. 4. Intellect—
Physiological aspects. I. Title.
QP376.K5   153   80-16410
ISBN 0-89116-202-X

*1989*

# the
# hedonistic
# neuron

**To Joni, Adam, and Zoe**

# contents

# preface

At the level of whole organisms it is commonly observed that animals pursue pleasure and avoid pain. At the level of the single neuron it is well known that the individual brain cell receives two classes of synaptic inputs: excitation and inhibition. What is the relationship between these two descriptions, one mentalistic and at an organismic level, the other physicalistic and at a neuronal level? Is there no simple relationship, as most neuroscientists would be likely to assume today? Have we described phenomena at two such vastly different levels and in such vastly different terms that the complexity and subtlety of their relationship will defy elucidation for some time to come? Or, to go to the other extreme, might their relationship be the simplest one conceivable? Namely, might excitation and inhibition represent, in elementary physical terms, one and the same thing that pleasure and pain represent in complex mental terms? But, at this point, can we even say precisely what we would mean by such questions? And even if we can, are not such questions simplistic to the point of being unproductive? This book seeks to demonstrate that we can say what we mean and that we will benefit from asking such questions.

The book examines a theory of brain function based on the postulate that neurons "seek" excitation and "avoid" inhibition, this goal being pursued within well-defined limits that preclude an epileptic outcome (except under pathological circumstances that, indeed, we know do arise). In the development of the theory, it will be seen that a plausible adaptive mechanism exists that can account, in mechanistic terms, for the postulated neuronal behavior. Also, .the notion of an excitation-seeking, inhibition-avoiding neuron will be shown to be consistent with experimentally observed neuronal behavior. Neuronal and cortical polarization studies, the mirror focus, and epileptic foci appear to be understandable in light of the proposed neuronal model. At a psychological level, habituation, dishabituation, classical and operant conditioning, and extinction can be shown to be straightforward consequences of a goal-seeking neuron like the kind proposed. None of this is to suggest that the validity of the proposed theory is demonstrated here. Far from it. Difficult experiments will have to be performed at the neuronal level to test the theory rigorously. Until these experiments are accomplished, the significance of the theory lies in its offering a fundamentally new view of brain function, a view that suggests alternative, and perhaps more productive, experiments.

The theory to be developed explains goal-seeking brain function in terms of goal-seeking neurons. It has been generally (and implicitly) assumed in the past that advanced (intelligent) goal-seeking brain function *emerges* from the interactions of non-goal-seeking neurons. Assuming such a passive, non-goal-seeking role for the neuron may not be valid. The single neuron is a remarkably complex and sophisticated cell and it may well play a more active role. Perhaps an analogy will help to make the point clear. Consider that goal-seeking social systems (such as the United States) would probably remain mysterious if we assumed that the people making up the social systems were non-goal-seeking in nature. There would probably be no way of explaining complex goal-seeking social system behavior (such as putting a person on the moon) in terms of the interactions of non-goal-seeking people. Are we any more likely to be successful in understanding goal-seeking nervous systems by assuming non-goal-seeking neurons? It remains to be seen, of course, but with the currently accepted approaches, theoretical progress has been slow. Thus, it is appropriate to consider alternative questions. A central question of brain research has been, "What is it that neurons *do* and how do they do it?" In Chapter 1, we will begin by asking

"What is it that neurons *want* and how do they get it?" (Clearly, it is not sufficient to discuss neuronal function in anthropo-morphic, teleological terms. For scientific purposes, such a view must be translated into a mechanistic theory that is subject to experimental tests. Accomplishing such a translation will be one of our objectives in the chapters that follow.)

A central question to be dealt with is that of how mental phenomena relate to physical phenomena. An identity theory of the mind-brain relationship, while widely accepted and probably correct, represents only a partial solution of the mind-body problem. From a theoretical standpoint, the need is to map the mind's more global, psychological, qualitative phenomena into the brain's more local, neurophysiological, and quantitative phenomena. Expressed differently, we would like to map such phenomena as sensations, emotions, and thoughts into electro-chemical events. In the theory to be developed, we will focus on pleasure and pain as mental phenomena and excitation and inhi-bition as physical phenomena to see if these mental and physical constructs can be simply related and, if so, what the implications are. In this way, we will come to see a possible relationship be-tween our internal description of reality (the only thing we can know directly) and reality itself.

*A. Harry Klopf*

# acknowledgments

This book grew out of research accomplished at the Air Force Cambridge Research Laboratories while I was on a National Research Council Postdoctoral Resident Research Associateship. I am most grateful to the National Research Council and the Air Force Cambridge Research Laboratories for the research opportunity that the postdoctoral appointment provided.

In addition to the essential institutional support just noted, I have benefited from the encouragement and constructive criticism of many individuals. While some of them do not agree with my conclusions, they have all helped to make this a better book. I want to thank especially Michael Arbib, Andy Barto, Hew Crane, Edmond Dewan, Gordy Globus, Earl Gose, Cecil Gwinn, Chuck Hendrix, Nick Herbert, Tony Mucciardi, Marshall Pease, Nico Spinelli, Rich Sutton, Rocco Urbano, and Dave Waltz. Most of all, I want to thank my wife, Joan, for her editing and encouragement during the writing of this monograph.

This book is a revised and updated version of Air Force Cambridge Research Laboratories Special Report Number 133 (AFCRL-72-0164), *Brain Function and Adaptive Systems—A Heterostatic Theory*, L. G. Hanscom Field, Bedford, Massachusetts, March 3, 1972 (DDC Report AD 742259).

Chapter 4, in revised form, appeared in a paper entitled "Goal-Seeking Systems from Goal-Seeking Components: Implications for AI," *Cognition and Brain Theory Newsletter*, Vol. 3, No. 2, 1979.

*A. Harry Klopf*

# abbreviations

| | |
|---|---|
| AI | Artificial Intelligence |
| CNS | Central Nervous System |
| CPU | Central Processing Unit |
| CR | Conditioned Response |
| CS | Conditioned Stimulus |
| I/O | Input/Output |
| IPSP | Inhibitory Postsynaptic Potential |
| LSH | Limbic System and Hypothalamus |
| LTM | Long-Term Memory |
| Ms | Milliseconds |
| MTRF | Midbrain and Thalamic Reticular Formation |
| NCS | Neural Conditioned Stimulus |
| NUS | Neural Unconditioned Stimulus |
| REM | Rapid Eye Movement |
| RF | Reticular Formation |
| STM | Short-Term Memory |
| UR | Unconditioned Response |
| US | Unconditioned Stimulus |

# the
# hedonistic
# neuron

# Chapter 1
# heterostasis

## 1.1 INTRODUCTION

A theory of intelligent adaptive systems is proposed in this and the following chapters. The theory offers a unifying framework within which the neurophysiological, psychological, and sociological properties of living adaptive systems can be understood. Furthermore, a new basis is suggested for the synthesis of machines possessing adaptive intelligence.

In this introductory chapter, the fundamental ideas underlying the theory are discussed. The proposed approach is compared with current conceptual frameworks for understanding brain function and the principal conclusions, to be developed more formally in subsequent chapters, are reviewed.

The theory originated with the belief that a number of similarities between social systems and nervous systems might be important from a theoretical standpoint. Both social and nervous systems may be viewed as networks, each constructed basically out of a single type of element. In the case of nervous systems, the neuron constitutes the network element or building block; in the case of social systems, the network elements are whole organisms. In both nervous and social systems, the network elements receive inputs from many other elements and likewise send their outputs to many others. Thus, both types of systems possess connectivity patterns exhibiting substantial convergence and divergence. Beyond these simple structural parallels are interesting similarities relating to information processing characteristics. Both social and nervous systems are adaptive; they acquire new forms of behavior as a function of experience. In both, memory and learning are distributed; information is not stored in a highly localized fashion. Both types of networks employ a redundant structure permitting them to function reliably despite the fact that individual elements are continually dying or malfunctioning. A measure of the plasticity of these systems is suggested by the fact that both can undergo extensive damage resulting in the permanent loss of large numbers of network elements (for example, severe head wounds in the case of nervous systems or large-scale bombing attacks during war in the case of social systems) and yet, after a period of time, lost functions can often be recovered by the surviving elements. Such an array of network properties is indeed remarkable. At least, most people find these properties impressive in the case of nervous systems. Social systems, exhibiting the same properties, inspire less awe because such networks are at least partially understood.

The question arises of whether our understanding of social networks can be applied to neural networks. Analogies between nervous and social systems may seem tenuous, but let us examine some of the possibilities. What kinds of mechanisms account for the adaptive powers of nervous and social systems? Where are the mechanisms located within the networks? Concerning the latter question, a plausible answer is that the fundamental adaptive mechanisms are localized within the individual elements, rather than that adaptation is an emergent global phenomenon appearing only in large assemblies of interacting elements. A corollary to this belief is the notion that the pattern of interconnections within a network is derived from each element's individual actions, each element forming connections based on local circumstances. In the case of a social system, the individual network elements (whole organisms) can be observed as they continually evolve new patterns of communication. It seems likely that neurons might carry out a similar process in the brain, producing new connectivity patterns as a function of experience.

For the purpose of further speculation, there is a simple way to restate the questions we are considering here. Two systems will be said to be equivalent ($\equiv$) if their adaptive mechanisms and the information processing characteristics growing out of these mechanisms are essentially similar. It is conjectured that from this system theoretic point of view, the following equivalence may be valid:

Nervous systems $\equiv$ social systems (1)

It is further conjectured that equivalence (1) is a consequence of the fundamental equivalence of the following two systems:

Neuron $\equiv$ whole organism (2)

Equivalence (2) seems to offer no insights whatever into neuronal function—until a philosophical notion is introduced into the analysis. Aristotle (384–322 B.C.) observed: "Happiness being found to be something final and self-sufficient, is the End at which all actions aim." Thus, a philosophical theory supplies a third equivalence:

Whole organism $\equiv$ hedonist (3)

From equivalences (2) and (3), a fourth equivalence is easily obtained and it provides the cornerstone of the theory to be proposed:

Neuron $\equiv$ hedonist (4)

Now, it is recognized that the above equivalences appear to be simplistic, at best. Being the product of loose, anthropomorphically oriented reasoning, there would appear to be little cause to pursue them further. However, the consequences of equivalence (4) have been found to be worthy of further investigation.

Unlike equivalence (2), equivalence (4) readily lends itself to an interpretation. Hedonism implies pleasurable and painful states, and there is a straightforward way of classifying neuronal states into two categories, these being the states of depolarization and hyperpolarization. Given the evident excitatory nature of pleasure and inhibitory nature of pain, the following equivalences suggest themselves for the neuron:

Depolarization ≡ pleasure                                            (5)

Hyperpolarization ≡ pain                                             (6)

One implication of these equivalences is that a neuron will seek to obtain excitation and to avoid inhibition. Does such a statement have a simple mechanistic interpretation? It does if one assumes, as many brain researchers currently do, that the efficacy of a synapse in causing a neuron to fire is a variable quantity, altered as a function of experience. Variable synaptic transmittances are then assumed to be the repository of learning and memory. Granting this assumption, a simple neuronal adaptive mechanism can be proposed by utilizing Skinner's (1938) framework of operant conditioning, this time in conjunction with the neuron instead of the whole animal. The idea is this. After a neuron fires, it waits for a few hundred milliseconds or more to see how it will be affected by the action it has taken. If it experiences further depolarization within a second or so, it increases the effectiveness of the excitatory synapses that led to its firing in the first place, thereby increasing the probability that it will fire the next time that some fraction of these synapses is active. If, however, the action of firing is followed within a second or so with the experience of hyperpolarization, the neuron then increases the effectiveness of those inhibitory synapses that were active when it fired. In this way, the probability of responding again to the input configuration has been diminished. Thus, it is suggested that the neuron, in effect, views excitation as reward and inhibition as punishment. A highly effective excitatory synapse, when active, "informs" the neuron that it should fire because, by doing so, it is likely to receive additional excitation. A highly effective inhibitory synapse, when active, "informs" the neuron that it had better not fire because, to do so, is likely to bring on additional inhibition. The effectiveness of a synapse, therefore, encodes a causal relation, providing predictive information concerning the consequences for the neuron if it fires when the synapse is active. It can be seen that the adaptive mechanism, over a period of time, will cause the neuron to behave so as to tend to maximize the amount of excitation and minimize the amount of inhibition being received.

The proposed neuronal model can be described in psychological terms. For a neuron, temporal and spatial configurations of active synapses represent conditioned stimuli (CS), firing represents a conditioned response (CR), and the excitation or inhibition that arrives during a limited period of time after firing constitutes the unconditioned stimulus (US). But if this is so, how does a neuron distinguish between an input configuration that represents a CS and one that represents a US? The answer may be that it does not. The neuronal US may simultaneously represent a CS with respect to signals that will arrive still later. At all times, neuronal inputs may be playing dual roles, representing conditioned stimuli with respect to near-future inputs and unconditioned stimuli with respect to recent-past inputs. This would permit an associative chaining of sequences of events.

Equivalence (4) would not have been considered as the basis for a brain theory (and, more generally, an adaptive network theory) had it not been for the support the resulting theory receives from the experimental literature of neurophysiology and psychology. Observations that appear to be relevant to learning mechanisms, obtained from neuronal and cortical polarization experiments and from the study of epileptic foci, are explained by the theory. Also, the theory provides explanations for the experimental results obtained in psychological studies of conditioning, habituation, extinction, and related phenomena. For these reasons, it was decided that a more rigorous development of the theory should be undertaken. This development begins in Chapter 2. The remainder of this chapter is devoted to a brief historical review, an introduction to the concept of heterostasis, and a summary of the main conclusions derived from the theory.

## 1.2  ASSUMPTIONS: PAST, PRESENT, AND PROPOSED

Let us define several types of systems and then note how our understanding of them has evolved. In doing this, we may come to see more clearly some of our assumptions as well as their origins.

We may define a *non-goal-seeking system* to be an open-loop system. It simply processes inputs and generates outputs. A *goal-seeking system*, on the other hand, utilizes feedback information to move toward or maintain a particular system state that is the goal. An *adaptive system* may be defined to be a system that modifies its own structure as a function of experience such that, over a period of time, the system's performance tends to improve relative to some criterion. An *adaptive network* is an adaptive system composed of (relatively) simple and homogeneous components functioning in a decentralized, highly parallel fashion.

As one way of viewing the evolution of our understanding of these systems, we may observe that the industrial revolution taught us a great deal about non-goal-seeking systems. More particularly, it is important to note that the industrial revolution taught us about non-goal-seeking systems composed of non-goal-seeking components. (A "component" here is any functional entity below the system level.) The cybernetic revolution that began in the 1940's has taught us the importance of *information* (as distinct from matter and energy) and the importance of feedback mechanisms. The result is a still rapidly increasing understanding of goal-seeking systems. These are largely, however, goal-seeking systems composed of non-goal-seeking components. Thus, goal-seeking in these systems is an emergent property. Also, these goal-seeking systems are generally non-adaptive. We may term them *control systems.* Further categories of systems can be envisioned and some of them have received very little attention. There is the category of goal-seeking systems composed of goal-seeking components. Still richer categories exist beyond this. Adaptive versions of goal-seeking systems are not well understood today; in fact, we have hardly made a beginning in this area.

It is interesting to consider where brains fall within this hierarchy of system types. Brains are both goal-seeking and adaptive. But what of the nature of their components, the neurons? It has generally been assumed that brains are goal-seeking systems composed of non-goal-seeking components. Some neuronal models that have been proposed could be interpreted as representing goal-seeking components, but only in a certain trivial sense. The Perceptron (Rosenblatt, 1957, 1960, 1962) is an example. A global reinforcer supplies inputs that are, in effect, direct orders to components to change input/output relations. However, without some kind of local reinforcement, as discussed below, it is not very meaningful to consider the component, itself, as having a goal.

Implicit assumptions concerning the nature of the components underlying brain function probably have a variety of roots. The industrial revolution taught us to think in terms of non-goal-seeking components and this habit probably carried over when we began to consider goal-seeking systems. Another reason for the disposition toward a non-goal-seeking view of the neuron may be that it is difficult to credit such interesting properties as goal-seeking to something that is very small. Most of us probably possess this strong prejudice associated with size. A neuron is barely visible to the naked eye. It is difficult to extend to the neuron much respect. It becomes easier, however, as one draws up close and observes the remarkably complex machinery that is contained within the single neuron, or any other cell for that matter. (For those who would like to further their appreciation of local mechanisms in living systems, Thomas (1974) provides a delightful nontheoretical discussion of *The Lives of a Cell*.)

If neurons are assumed to function as non-goal-seeking components, then goal-seeking brain function must be viewed as an emergent phenomenon. Can such a view lead to explanations for memory, learning and, more generally, intelligence? So far, such a view has not yielded understanding. Certain cybernetic analyses of neural nets (see Griffith, 1962, 1963; Uttley, 1966, 1975; Wilkins, 1970; Klopf, 1972, 1975) suggest a possible reason: Particular kinds of local feedback mechanisms that have been absent from most brain models may be crucial to the emergence of intelligence. The implication of the cited neural net studies is that intelligent brain function can perhaps only be understood if it is assumed that *the single neuron is a goal-seeking system in its own right.* This postulate applies, of course, only to plastic (i.e., adaptive) neurons. For the purposes of this discussion, neurons with fixed input/output relations need not be considered.

In taking the notion of goal-seeking down to the level of the single neuron, it should be noted that it might be possible to go even further. However, an infinite regression is not anticipated. It seems likely that during the evolutionary process, goal-seeking phenomena first emerged at the level of the single cell or at a functional level not much lower than this. For example, there appears to be no basis for associating goal-seeking behavior with such entities as atoms or molecules.

It should also be made clear that the neuronal goal being proposed here has to do with neuronal inputs, not outputs. Thus, it is not being suggested that the goal of the single neuron is to fire, but rather to obtain excitation and avoid inhibition. Regardless of how it may appear, goal-seeking systems always manipulate outputs for the sake of controlling inputs. The distinction is an important one, as Powers (1973) has shown in *Behavior: The Control of Perception*.

While neurons have usually been assumed to be non-goal-seeking, whole brains have been assumed to be pursuing the goal of homeostasis. These kinds of assumptions, where basic components are assumed to be non-goal-seeking and whole systems are assumed to be homeostatic, are probably appropriate for plants, perhaps also for animals on the low end of the phylogenetic scale and for certain large bureaucracies. However, as intelligence begins to emerge in complex networks, it will be hypothesized here that a new goal begins to manifest itself. Homeostasis becomes a subgoal (albeit a crucial one) and a new goal takes over: *it is hypothesized that intelligence in complex systems is a concomitant of a striving for a maximal condition*. We may term this maximal condition *heterostasis*.

Is there any evidence to support this hypothesis? We can broadly consider this question here in the introduction. More specific aspects of the question will be addressed in subsequent chapters.

Both from phylogenetic and ontogenetic standpoints, as intelligence in living systems increases, the amount of apparent homeostatic behavior exhibited decreases, culminating in the case of humans with behavior that seems often to be decidedly nonhomeostatic. While it is true that any behavior including, for example, volunteering to go the moon, can be and has been interpreted as being homeostatic, such ad hocism is not convincing. While homeostasis makes sense as the goal of the autonomic nervous system, the same cannot be said for the somatic nervous system. The assumption that homeostasis is the goal of the somatic nervous system has not led to understanding. It will be suggested here that the goal of the somatic nervous system (the substrate of intelligence) is to obtain reward and to avoid punishment or, put another way, to maximize the difference between the amounts of reward and punishment obtained. And this need not remain an ill-defined statement, as it has been in the past. The framework that will be developed in the following chapters opens up the possibility of mapping the broad mental variables of pleasure and pain along with the broad behavioral variables of positive and negative reinforcement into the specific physiological variables of excitation and inhibition.

## 1.3 HETEROSTASIS: A MAXIMAL CONDITION

The analysis and synthesis of intelligent adaptive systems is the objective of the theory proposed in this and the following chapters. The fundamental postulate of the theory is discussed in this section. Chapters 2 and 3 further develop and test the theory, utilizing evidence from neurophysiology and psychology. Cybernetic issues, in general, are considered in Chapter 4.

One general theory concerned with adaptive systems already exists. The theory is based on a concept proposed in 1859 by Claude Bernard. The concept is now referred to as homeostasis, a term introduced by Walter Cannon (1929). Homeostasis refers to the condition of a system in which a set of "essential variables" has assumed steady state values compatible with the system's continued ability to function. Essential variables are defined by Ashby (1960) to be those "which are closely related to survival and which are closely linked dynamically." A theory that evolved from the concept of homeostasis suggests that this condition is the goal of all animal behavior. Ashby (1960) has concluded, for example, that homeostasis is the goal of "a great deal, if not all, of the normal human adult's behavior." Young (1966) has stated a similar conclusion: "Brains are the computers of homeostats and the essence of homeostats is that they maintain a steady state. Put in another way, the most important fact about living things is that they remain alive."

It will be proposed here that homeostasis is not the primary goal of more phylogenetically advanced living systems; rather, that it is a secondary or subgoal. It is suggested that the primary goal is a condition which, following the example of Cannon (1929), will be termed heterostasis. An organism will be said to be in a condition of heterostasis with respect to a specific internal variable when that variable has been maximized. Heterostasis, as the term itself suggests, is not associated with a steady-state condition. In general, the internal variable to be maximized will have an upper limit that changes as environmental constraints change. Therefore, even if heterostasis is continuously maintained by an organism, a steady-state condition with respect to the internal variable will not result. Furthermore, if the maximal condition does turn out, in special cases, also to be a steady-state condition, it will still be useful to distinguish it as a maximal condition because, in general, the pursuit of such a condition (goal) involves different kinds of adaptive mechanisms than does the pursuit of a steady-state condition.

The belief that homeostasis provides a sufficient basis for explaining the behavior of living systems is widespread. It is true that homeostatic variables do appear at all levels of organization of living systems, beginning at the level of the single cell and extending through the levels of the whole organism and the society. However, homeostatic variables alone appear to provide an incomplete description. In more advanced organisms, at every level of organization, one also sees evidence for heterostatic variables and, in fact, the evidence to be reviewed in subsequent chapters suggests that heterostasis is the ultimate goal. In general, it appears that within the domain of the autonomic nervous system, regulation is accomplished with innate homeostatic mechanisms. Within the domain of the somatic nervous system, learning appears to be accomplished with heterostatic mechanisms.

Maintenance of the condition of heterostasis is not necessary for survival, in contrast to the maintenance of homeostasis which is an essential condition for life. In fact, with respect to heterostasis, it will be seen that advanced living systems infrequently or never achieve the condition. For this reason, it is appropriate to define a heterostatic system as one that seeks (moves toward) a maximal condition while not necessarily ever achieving it.

To some, it may appear paradoxical that heterostasis is hypothesized to be the primary goal of advanced living systems, while it is further suggested that this condition is *not* essential to the maintenance of life. Homeostasis, on the other hand, is here hypothesized to be a *secondary* goal and yet it is essential to life. This apparent paradox will dissolve if one is careful not to assume that the maintenance of life is necessarily the primary goal of all living systems. In a Darwinian process, while survival is clearly a constraint, it need not be the goal. Indeed, the emergence of intelligence (as a result of its survival value) may only be possible for organisms that evolve a goal structure beyond that of the homeostat. Homeostats may simply be too passive to become intelligent.

## 1.4  CONCLUSIONS: IMPLICATIONS
## OF A HETEROSTATIC THEORY

In this introductory chapter, we have been discussing, in part, the question of images, the kinds of images that guide our thinking. If we are to understand intelligence in living systems, it seems that our image of brain function may have to change radically. The view that brains are collections of bureaucrat-like neurons that simply process information and adapt in support of global goals may not be tenable. A more promising image may be that of goal-seeking, adaptive neurons actively participating in establishing a consensus—a consensus of neural activity that, first of all, supports the neuron's own needs. That this emerging consensus may also be something more, namely, the phenomenon of "intelligence," is not of direct consequence for the single neuron. The view that will be emphasized here is that the single adaptive neuron can only pursue its own goal and then let intelligence emerge as a by-product, if it will. (If it does not, of course, the Darwinian process may have something to say about it.)

A crucial aspect of the theory developed in subsequent

chapters is the idea that neuronal inputs, in general, are reinforcing; excitation constitutes reward and inhibition constitutes punishment. This leads to the view of a goal-seeking, adaptive neuronal substrate that can support intelligence, in part, through sheer size. With an emphasis on local mechanisms, a vast, decentralized substrate becomes possible. Consider that a typical neuron has, perhaps, ten thousand synaptic inputs (Haug, 1972). If many or most of these inputs are functioning as reinforcing feedback loops, then it can be seen that the adaptive neuron is embedded in its environment in an especially rich kind of way. The human nervous system contains, perhaps, $10^{12}$ neurons and most of them may be plastic. Therefore, at the neuronal level, human brain function may involve the operation of something approaching $10^{16}$ reinforcing feedback loops. If the human brain is embedded in its environment in this way, one may begin to see how the environment comes to be internalized so effectively. With each of approximately $10^{12}$ neurons exploring, in parallel, the consequences of activating something like $10^4$ reinforcing feedback loops, it becomes plausible that such a neuronal substrate could develop into a vast microscopic, nonlinguistic knowledge base. In the case of an individual, only after a number of years of environmental programming can more global, more macroscopic, often linguistically oriented, kinds of information processing tasks be successfully learned. Thus, we can begin to see how the more advanced macroscopic capabilities associated with intelligence are, perhaps, built on the foundation of an immense microscopic knowledge base that would seem to be an essential first step. This view may be contrasted with that assumed in current artificial intelligence (AI) research, in which an attempt is made to proceed directly to a more advanced capability that is psychologically and linguistically oriented. The AI approach appears to have an advantage in bypassing the time consuming first step of establishing a more microscopic knowledge base. However, as will be discussed in Chapter 4, there is no evidence yet that the current AI approach is a viable strategy if the objective is to obtain highly intelligent systems.

By way of providing an overview, it may be helpful at this point to summarize the conclusions that will be developed in subsequent chapters. The overall conclusion is that intelligent brain function can be understood in terms of nested hierarchies of heterostatic goal-seeking adaptive loops, beginning at the level of the single neuron and extending upward to the level of the whole brain. More specifically, it is suggested that:

1. The primary goal of more advanced animals, including humans, is the achievement of a maximal condition, not the achievement of a steady-state condition. In their highest level functions, intelligent animals are not homeostats, they are heterostats (a heterostat is defined to be a system that seeks a maximal condition). The variable to be maximized is the amount of neuronal polarization being experienced. The amount of polarization is defined to be equal to the amount of depolarization (hypothesized to be one and the same thing as pleasure) minus the amount of hyperpolarization (hypothesized to be one and the same thing as pain). The heterostatic nature of more advanced (intelligent) animals derives from the heterostatic nature of their controlling neurons.

2. Heterostatic nervous systems are so structured that homeostasis is a necessary but not sufficient condition for the maintenance of heterostasis. Intelligent animals vigorously pursue homeostasis at "lower levels," although it is not their primary goal. That homeostasis is a *sub*goal suggests that survival may not be as central a concern of living systems as has generally been assumed.

3. Experimental results obtained in neuronal and cortical polarization studies and the results obtained in the study of epileptic foci can be explained in terms of whether a depolarizing or hyperpolarizing bias is imposed on the neurons involved. A depolarizing bias is rewarding and causes the effectiveness of recently active excitatory synapses to increase. A hyperpolarizing bias is punishing and causes the effectiveness of recently active inhibitory synapses to increase. Epilepsy is a progressive disease because established epileptic foci continue to deliver polarizing biases to normal neural tissue. This tissue, in turn, undergoes adaptation in response to the imposed bias and becomes hyper- or hypoactive, depending on the polarity of the imposed bias.

4. Habituation, dishabituation, classical conditioning, operant conditioning, and extinction are phenomena that can be

understood in terms of the neuronal adaptive response to depolarizing or hyperpolarizing reinforcement. Also of importance in understanding the mechanisms underlying habituation are feed-forward and recurrent inhibition as well as the existence of long-duration IPSP neurons. The mechanisms underlying habituation and extinction are fundamentally the same.

5. The solution to the mind-body problem is an identity theory. A neuron undergoing depolarization *is* elementary pleasure; a neuron undergoing hyperpolarization *is* elementary pain. The subjective experience of pleasure or pain is identical to the objective event of neurons undergoing depolarization or hyperpolarization, respectively. Pleasure and pain provide the single bidirectional dimension necessary to analyze mental phenomena. Pleasure and pain are much more fundamental and broader concepts than previously assumed. Complex forms of pleasure and pain (that is, the full range of possible mental states) are one and the same as complex spatial configurations of depolarizing and hyperpolarizing neurons. Each configuration corresponds to a particular mental state. The neurons which constitute the dynamic configuration corresponding to the "mind" are those of the midbrain and thalamic reticular formation (MTRF). Our "mind" is aware of other neural structures only to the extent that their outputs impinge on the MTRF. Pleasurable mental states result when depolarizing neurons are more prevalent in the MTRF. Painful mental states result when hyperpolarizing neurons are more prevalent. The exact mental state depends upon the exact configuration of depolarizing and hyperpolarizing neurons within the MTRF. The mental states corresponding to feeling tone, sensation, and ideation result when the principal inputs to the MTRF are supplied by the limbic system and hypothalamus, sensory cortex, or nonsensory-nonmotor cortex, respectively.

6. The global organization of the brain can be understood in terms of three major subsystems: The midbrain and thalamic reticular formation (MTRF), the limbic system and hypothalamus (LSH), and the neocortex. The MTRF, by virtue of its unique position, has become the command and control center and the seat of conscious awareness. (This conclusion, which runs contrary to prevailing opinion today, is reconciled with

split-brain and other evidence in Chapter 3.) The MTRF seeks to obtain excitation and to avoid inhibition. Its sources for both types of signal are the sensory and pain fibers, the LSH, and the neocortex. In general, sensory fibers are excitatory with respect to the MTRF; pain fibers are inhibitory with respect to the MTRF. The LSH, utilizing the innate mechanisms of its reinforcement centers, delivers generalized excitation or inhibition to the MTRF, depending on whether the MTRF's decisions are leading toward or away from homeostasis. Also, the innate mechanisms corresponding to drive centers permit the LSH to make decisions concerning more specific actions to be taken to maintain homeostasis. The neocortex provides input/ output functions and memory for the MTRF. It preprocesses incoming information, provides storage, and elaborates on the MTRF's motor commands. Curiosity is a manifestation of the fundamental drive for depolarizing stimuli. (Novel stimuli must be sought because the habituation mechanism renders repetitive stimuli ineffective.) The "attention" mechanism and the facili- tation of limited cortical areas by the MTRF are synonymous. Facilitation delivered by the MTRF to the cortex is positively reinforcing and we, therefore, remember that to which we attend, while not remembering that to which we do not attend. Recall occurs when the MTRF is driven by its variety of inputs into a state approximating one it has been in before. It then sends a signal configuration to the cortex like that which it sent out before. The result is that the MTRF facilitates cortical memories laid down during the previous experience. The MTRF becomes aware of these memories when the outputs of the facilitated cortical neurons reach the MTRF. Memory is that information acquired with cortical reinforcement supplied by the MTRF attention mechanism; learning is that information acquired with reinforcement supplied by sensory, pain fiber, or LSH activity.

7. Not only neurons, assemblies of neurons, and whole nervous systems are heterostats, the same is true for families, neighborhoods, cities, regions, and nations.

8. Historically, there have been two approaches to adaptive networks (or, more narrowly, neural networks). One approach is to employ an *association model* of the neuron, where adaptation

is a function of correlation measures between a neuron's inputs and output. Hebb (1949) initiated detailed analyses of this type of model. An alternative approach is to employ a *reinforcement model* of the neuron, where adaptation is a function of reinforcement signals received by the neuron some time after the occurrence of the behavior to be modified. The Perceptron (Rosenblatt, 1957, 1962) is the best known example in this category. If one adopts a reinforcement model of the neuron, there are still two alternatives to be considered. In the case of *restricted reinforcement models*, of which the Perceptron is typical, only one or two neuronal inputs are reinforcing, these originating usually in some global reinforcement mechanism. In the case of *generalized reinforcement models*, all (or at least many) inputs to the neuron are reinforcing, with the reinforcing signals originating sometimes locally and sometimes globally. The heterostat is an example of a generalized reinforcement model. Restricted reinforcement models, as well as association models, were widely investigated in the 1950s and 1960s, but this research did not lead to conclusive results, at least for the general case of multilayered adaptive networks. Generalized reinforcement models offer a new approach to brain theory and adaptive network research.

9. Artificial intelligence research has been importantly shaped by the (implicit) assumption of a non-goal-seeking view of the neuron, the (temporary) assumption of a conventional digital computer as the hardware substrate for intelligence and the (seemingly expedient) assumption that one should proceed directly to research at psychological and linguistic levels, foregoing investigations of what might be an appropriate substrate at something like the neuronal level. These assumptions and some others to which they have led appear questionable with respect to the long term AI goal of developing highly intelligent systems.

# Chapter 2
# neurophysiology

To summarize the neuronal model as thus far discussed, neurons seek to maximixe the amount of depolarization and to minimize the amount of hyperpolarization they are experiencing. A neuron accomplishes this by modifying the effectiveness of its synapses after impulse generation. If impulse generation is followed by further depolarization, the effectiveness of recently active excitatory synapses is increased. If hyperpolarization follows impulse generation, the effectiveness of recently active inhibitory synapses is increased. "Recently active synapses" are those that contributed the excitation or inhibition that was effective during the generation of the impulses. "To seek a goal" and "to move, by means of feedback, toward a particular system state" are equivalent expressions in this discussion. The heterostatic model of the neuron will be more precisely defined in Section 2.1. A comparison with alternative neuronal models will be accomplished in Chapter 4.

## 2.1 THE NEURONAL MODEL

### 2.1.1 Neuronal Heterostasis

It will be helpful to define the heterostatic model of the neuron in mathematical terms. For nonmathematical readers, it may be noted that the mathematics presented in this section is not essential to a general understanding of the theory, although it would still be desirable to read the accompanying text, noting the alternative definitions of the heterostatic variable, $\mu$.

A neuron will be viewed as receiving $n$ numbered synaptic inputs, each of which delivers a series of action potentials. The frequency of arrival of impulses at the $i$th synapse will be represented as the input intensity, $f_i(t)$. This measure of frequency reflects the activity of the synapse at time, $t$. Also, for each synapse, there will be a weight, $w_i$, representing the synaptic transmittance or effectiveness associated with the frequency, $f_i(t)$. Weights are constrained to be positive in the case of excitatory inputs and negative in the case of inhibitory inputs. The weights are postulated to be the repository of learning and memory and, therefore, they vary with time according to the experience of the organism. Also, a weight in this model reflects an input's effectiveness as a function of the location of the synapse on the soma or within the dendritic field.

The computation that a neuron performs in "deciding" whether to fire consists of a spatial and temporal summation of the weighted inputs followed by a thresholding operation. That is to say, the neuron generates an action potential only if the following relationship holds:

$$\sum_{i=1}^{n} w_i(t) f_i(t) \geqslant \theta(t_o) \tag{7}$$

where $n$ = the number of synaptic inputs

$\quad w_i(t)$ = the synaptic transmittance associated with the $i$th input; positive and negative weights correspond to excitation and inhibition, respectively.

$\quad f_i(t)$ = a frequency measure of the input intensity at the $i$th synapse

$\quad \theta(t_o)$ = the neuronal threshold

$\quad\quad t$ = time

$\quad\quad t_o$ = the time elapsed since the generation of the last action potential

In Inequality (7), the spatial variations in the effectiveness of the inputs are reflected in the weights. Temporal variations are incorporated into the measure of frequency employed in arriving at the value of $f_i(t)$. $\theta$ must be a function of $t_o$ in order to account for the experimentally observed variation in the threshold during the absolute and relative refractory periods.

The variable that is maximized when a system achieves the condition of heterostasis is denoted by $\mu$ and termed the *heterostatic variable.* Neuronal heterostasis is defined as the condition in which the amount of polarization being experienced by a neuron is maximal, relative to constraints imposed by the neuron's environment and adaptive mechanism. *De*polarization and *hyper*polarization represent the positive and negative components, respectively, of polarization. More precisely, a neuron is said to be in a condition of heterostasis for the time interval ranging from $t$ to $t + \tau$ if its synaptic transmittances are such as to maximize the quantity, $\mu_1{}^{t,t+\tau}$:

$$\mu_1{}^{t,t+\tau} = D_{t,t+\tau} - H_{t,t+\tau} \tag{8}$$

$$\mu_1{}^{t,t+\tau} = \int_t^{t+\tau} [v_p(t) - v_r]\, dt - \int_t^{t+\tau} [v_n(t) - v_r]\, dt \tag{9}$$

$$\mu_1{}^{t,t+\tau} = \int_t^{t+\tau} [v(t) - v_r]\, dt \tag{10}$$

where $D_{t,t+\tau}$ = the amount of depolarization experienced during the interval, $t$ to $t + \tau$

$H_{t,t+\tau}$ = the amount of hyperpolarization experienced during the interval, $t$ to $t + \tau$

$v(t)$ = the potential difference across the neuronal membrane

$v_r$ = the resting potential of the neuron

$v_p(t) = v(t)$ if $v(t) \geqslant v_r$, otherwise $v_p(t) = v_r$

$v_n(t) = v(t)$ if $v(t) \leqslant v_r$, otherwise $v_n(t) = v_r$

In Eq. (8), $\mu$ is subscripted in order to distinguish this approach to the definition of neuronal heterostasis from another presented below.

Constraints imposed by the neuron's adaptive process (not yet detailed) make the maximization of $\mu_1$ an unattainable goal, in general. The definition is offered, however, because it represents a useful way of specifying the condition towards which a neuron moves (within a stable environment) and in this sense does represent the neuronal goal. An alternative definition of neuronal heterostasis, suggesting a condition that is more nearly attainable, is that which defines the goal to be the maximization of $\mu_2$ :

$$\mu_2 = E\left[\sum_{i=1}^{n} w_i(t)f_i(t)\right] = E[\alpha(t) - \beta(t)] \tag{11}$$

where

$$\alpha(t) = \sum_{i=1}^{m} w_i(t)f_i(t) \tag{12}$$

$$\beta(t) = -\sum_{i=m+1}^{n} w_i(t)f_i(t) \tag{13}$$

$[1 \leqslant i \leqslant m]$ = the range of the numbered excitatory synapses and $[(m + 1) \leqslant i \leqslant n]$ = the range of the numbered inhibitory synapses.

$E[x]$ refers to the expected or average value of $x$, in this case computed for the set of all input configurations that the neuron may receive. If $\mu_2$ is to be maximized, the weights, $w_i(t)$, must be adjusted such that the average difference between the amount of excitation, $\alpha(t)$, and the amount of inhibition, $\beta(t)$, that is received is maximized. To the extent that $\alpha(t)$ and $\beta(t)$ are independent variables, the following equation holds:

$$\begin{aligned} \max(\mu_2) &= \max\{E[\alpha(t) - \beta(t)]\} \\ &= \max\{E[\alpha(t)]\} - \min\{E[\beta(t)]\} \end{aligned} \tag{14}$$

Equation (14) suggests that although neurons may appear to be maximizing the amount of excitation and minimizing the amount of inhibition received, they may actually be seeking to maximize the difference between these two quantities.

### 2.1.2  Adaptation

Having suggested that neurons seek depolarization and avoid hyperpolarization (within certain limits), the question that must now be considered is whether there is a plausible adaptive process that will produce such behavior. It should be noted that this discussion will pertain only to neurons possessing plasticity. The possibly substantial fraction of nonadaptive neurons within nervous systems are of interest here only in that they represent part of the environment of the adaptive neurons.

Let us consider two possible ways in which $\mu$ might be made to increase. A trivial way is to set the inhibitory weights equal to zero and the excitatory weights at their upper limits (which are assumed to be finite). Alternatively, with the proper adjustment of the weights, the firing of the neuron can be made to occur at such times as to result in the frequency of arrival of depolarizing input configurations being maximized and the frequency of arrival of hyperpolarizing input configurations being minimized. Only the latter possibility can provide a basis for learning (and survival). Therefore, the adaptive process to be proposed employs the second approach and excludes the first.

When a neuron fires, the output signal may be viewed as being fed back to the input side of the neuron via a variety of channels (see Figure 1). One channel involves the remainder of the nervous system and constitutes neural feedback. Another channel provides information from the remainder of the organism's internal environment. The third channel is the external environmental feedback loop. The number of individual feedback loops available to a neuron can be very large. A Purkinje cell in the cerebellum, for example, receives about 200,000 excitatory synaptic inputs from the system of "parallel" fibers (Eccles, 1969a). Large cortical pyramidal cells may receive more than 10,000 excitatory inputs (Eccles, 1966). It is therefore possible for a neuron to receive a tremendous variety of input

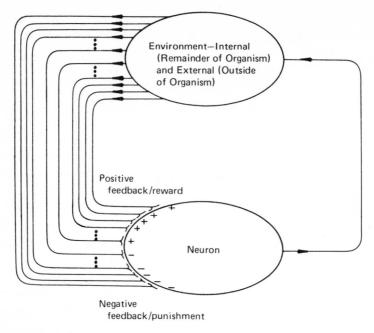

**FIGURE 1.** Relationship of a heterostatic neuron to its internal and external environment.

combinations, indicating that a neuron's view of the world may be a highly varied and complex one.

It will be assumed that neurons utilize the feedback loops in "deciding" to which input configurations they will respond. Specifically, it is proposed that neurons will be more likely to respond again to stimulus configurations that led to firing if the neuronal response, when fed back, results in further depolarization. However, if the feedback arrives in the form of inhibition, the neuron eventually ceases to respond to the input configuration preceding the inhibition. The following postulated mechanism will produce these neuronal behavioral changes by altering synaptic transmittances according to three rules:

1. When a neuron fires, all of its excitatory and inhibitory synapses that were active during the summation of potentials leading to the response are eligible to undergo changes in their transmittances.

2. The transmittance of an eligible *excitatory* synapse

increases if the generation of the action potential is followed by further depolarization, that is,

$$\left| \sum_{i=1}^{m} w_i(t) f_i(t) \right| > \left| \sum_{i=m+1}^{n} w_i(t) f_i(t) \right| \tag{15}$$

for a limited time interval after the response.

3. The transmittance of an eligible *inhibitory* synapse increases, that is, it becomes more negative, if the generation of an action potential is followed by hyperpolarization, that is,

$$\left| \sum_{i=1}^{m} w_i(t) f_i(t) \right| < \left| \sum_{i=m+1}^{n} w_i(t) f_i(t) \right| \tag{16}$$

for a limited time interval after the response. This process whereby synaptic transmittances are altered so as to increase $\mu$ will be termed *heterostatic adaptation*.

It is useful to define this adaptive process in terms of the psychological variables of operant conditioning, both for the purpose of further clarifying the mechanism and because of the relevance of a psychologically oriented definition to later considerations. In the interest of simplifying the discussion, incoming neuronal stimuli will be viewed as arriving at discrete time intervals. We can then discuss a stimulus, $s_t$, consisting of some configuration of excitatory and inhibitory inputs, followed by the stimulus, $s_{t+1}$, etc. Heterostatic adaptation may then be viewed as follows. A neuronal input configuration, $s_t$, which causes the neuron to fire, will be termed a neural conditioned stimulus (NCS). The stimuli, $s_{t+1}$ through $s_{t+j}$, received by the neuron for a limited time interval after the NCS, constitute the neural unconditioned stimulus (NUS). The NUS is rewarding if $s_{t+1}$ through $s_{t+j}$ generally result in depolarization, and punishing if these inputs generally result in hyperpolarization.

Having broadly outlined the process of heterostatic adaptation, speculation can now be offered concerning some of the detailed aspects of the mechanism. For example, in Pavlovian conditioning, the most effective US is one that arrives approximately 400 ms after the CS (see review by Russell, 1966). A US that arrives sooner or later than 400 ms after the CS has a reduced reinforcing effect. The reinforcing effect decreases to zero with (a) simultaneous occurrence of the CS and the US or (b) with a CS-US interval that exceeds a few seconds. It is hypothesized that these temporal relationships between the CS and US reflect similar temporal relationships between the NCS and NUS.

It seems reasonable to expect that synapses mediating an NUS cannot undergo transmittance changes in response to that NUS, even if these synapses also mediated the NCS. Synapses that mediated *only* the NCS will undergo transmittance changes if the NUS (utilizing other synapses) follows within no more than a few seconds. In consideration of these factors and those noted in the paragraph above, it is hypothesized that a synapse must be inactive for about 400 ms in order to be maximally reinforced. This model does not rule out the possibility of an input configuration to a neuron serving as an NUS relative to a preceding input configuration and serving as an NCS relative to a future input configuration. The proposed mechanism that prevents a synapse from being modified if it mediates both the NCS and NUS will be termed *zerosetting*.

The motivation for introducing zerosetting in the model is to prevent an input configuration from being reinforced simply by repetition. If reinforcement could occur due to repetition alone, behavioral patterns could then be established without regard for their consequences. If such an undesirable feature is to be avoided, it is concluded that neuronal reinforcement must result from the interaction of distinct subsets of synapses. In some cases, it may turn out that zerosetting is accomplished by having specialized synapses that mediate only the NCS or the NUS, depending, perhaps, on whether the synapse is located on a dendrite or on the soma. If some synapses are specialized to this extent, then the transmittances of NUS-mediating synapses might not have to be modifiable.

It is hypothesized that the magnitude of an adaptive weight change, $\Delta w_i$, is not only a function of the delay between the NCS and the various portions of the NUS but is also a function of the magnitude of the polarization occurring throughout the effective reinforcement interval. Thus, mildly depolarizing or hyperpolarizing reinforcing signals accomplish lesser alterations in the synaptic transmittances than do stronger signals. This relationship would explain the greater extent of learning and the more vivid memories that result when an animal is highly aroused. More will be said about this in Chapter 3.

It should be noted that since the NUS is distributed over a time interval measuring up to perhaps 4 seconds in duration (see review by Russell, 1966), it will sometimes consist of a mix of depolarizing and hyperpolarizing input configurations. Whether an NUS positively or negatively reinforces, therefore, will depend on the relative amounts of each type of signal that are present and also on their arrival times during the 4-second interval.

A neuron must compute two functions; these will be designated as the *I/O function* and the adaptation or *α-function*. The former refers to the computation of the axonal output and the latter to the computation of the synaptic transmittance changes.

The extent of polarization of a neuron will be denoted by $\Sigma$. At the resting potential, $\Sigma$ will be defined to be equal to zero. Positive and negative values of $\Sigma$ will correspond to depolarized and hyperpolarized neuronal states, respectively.

In the heterostatic model of the neuron, $\Sigma$ plays a dual role. In the computation of the I/O function, the value of $\Sigma$ relative to the neuronal threshold determines whether the neuron will fire. In the case of the α-function, the value of $\Sigma$ determines whether the neuron is being rewarded or punished. Further, the amount of synaptic transmittance change, as noted above, is hypothesized to be approximately proportional to the absolute value of $\Sigma$, that is,

$$\Delta w_i \cong k|\Sigma| \tag{17}$$

where $k$ = constant.

The dual role of $\Sigma$ suggests a characteristic to be observed in nervous systems. The computations of the I/O and the α-function might, at times, interfere with one another because both utilize the same parameter. When the reinforcement centers (to be discussed in Chapter 3) deliver substantial excitatory or inhibitory reinforcement to a neuron, this will alter $\Sigma$ in a way that may be appropriate relative to transmittance modification but inappropriate relative to the current I/O computations. Seemingly similar kinds of interference can be observed with people. The experience of substantial positive or negative reinforcement can significantly alter a person's performance. For example, when people experience great disappointments, their behavior may become quite inappropriate, at least temporarily. Our hypothesis suggests that the punishing signals have, in effect, elevated neuronal thresholds by decreasing $\Sigma$. On the other hand, the experience of strong positive (excitatory) reinforcement can render a person incapable of complex information processing for a period of time. The reinforcement, in effect, lowers neuronal thresholds by increasing $\Sigma$. This is evidenced by hyperexcitability, which is usually incompatible with activities requiring a high degree of concentration. However, these effects should, themselves, be subject to reinforcement, and we would, therefore, expect to observe their reduction with experience.

### 2.1.3 Properties of the Model

It might appear that a heterostatic neuron, because it is continually seeking excitation, would eventually fire all the time, yielding a convulsion as the final brain state. The neuronal model proposed here, however, will not lead to convulsions, except under certain pathological conditions that do, in fact, lead to epilepsy (see Section 2.2.2). Under normal conditions, a convulsive state will not develop because a neuron's pursuit of excitation will, in general, be checked by the neuron's avoidance of inhibition, thus providing an effective balance. Neurons learn to fire in response to some inputs, but not to fire in response to others. In each case, it depends on what the past experience was with the particular subset of synapses that are presently active. If firing in the past yielded reward (i.e., additional excitation), then the excitatory synapses within the subset will have become increasingly effective and the neuron will more likely fire now. However, if firing in the past yielded punishment (inhibition), then the inhibitory synapses within the same subset will have become increasingly effective and the neuron will more likely not fire now.

The situation at the level of the single neuron may mirror the situation at the level of the whole organism. If, within a social system, negative feedback (pain) were somehow removed, a social analog of a convulsion would probably ensue. "Mob psychology" may be an example of such a phenomenon.

Another apparent problem with the proposed model is that it may seem as though the heterostatic neuron will be adapting continuously, thereby preventing any stable behavior patterns from emerging. Actually, this is unlikely because, in the detailed specification of the model, one sees that exacting constraints must be satisfied before adaptation can occur. Most learning, then, will consist of adjustments that amount to progressively finer tuning.

Another question of potential concern is whether synapses will "saturate" with continued reinforcement. That is to say, excitatory and inhibitory synapses might tend toward maximum efficacy if extended reinforcement occurs. However, if this condition arises in nervous systems, this would not necessarily affect adaptive neuronal function adversely. Learning may amount to the selection of *which* excitatory and inhibitory synapses are highly effective within the nervous system, not *how* effective they are to be. With perhaps $10^{16}$ variable synapses to select from, there may be no shortage. It is interesting to consider, for example, that it would be possible for the adaptive process of the brain to modify a billion synaptic transmittances every second for an average human lifetime without ever having to modify the same synapse twice. (This measure of the information coding capacity of the human brain provides an upper bound in that every synaptic transmittance is assumed to be modifiable, which is probably not the case.) Learning through practice then may refine the performance of a motor act simply through the successive involvement of new excitatory and inhibitory synapses, not through the fine tuning of already adapted ones.

Some questions regarding the heterostatic model of the neuron cannot be answered at this time, but the questions should be noted, nonetheless. Does the entire neuron act as a single heterostat as we have assumed, or do limited areas of the soma and dendritic field act independently of one another from the standpoint of adaptation? For example, could it be that recently active synapses are reinforced only by other active synapses in the immediate area rather than by synapses anywhere on the neuron?

It seems likely that some neurons are nonadaptive, realizing I/O relations that are forever fixed. If so, such neurons represent permanent constraints for the adaptive portion of the nervous system. Likewise, some of the synapses of adaptive neurons may not possess variable transmittances; this property may be reserved for certain specialized synapses. There is also the question of the role of nonsynaptic (electrotonic) neuronal connections. Do such connections possess a variable nature that can be utilized in memory and learning in a fashion similar to that of the variable synapses, or do they represent fixed initial conditions and perpetual constraints for the adaptive neuron? Certain more general questions need also to be considered. If only more advanced organisms are heterostats, at what point along the phylogenetic scale do homeostatic organisms start shading into heterostatic organisms? Because the genetic apparatus of neuronal cells is free of the responsibilities of reproduction (i.e., CNS cells do not regenerate), does this apparatus become available to encode modified transmittance values and then insure that these values are maintained? If so, might the recovery of function observed in retrograde amnesia, for instance, result from a DNA-directed repair process in which transmittances are reset to the values they had before injury? Further, might the sequence of transmittance values that originally occurred be approximated during the recovery process (a mnemonic version of ontogeny recapitulating phylogeny), thereby explaining the order in which memories return?

## 2.2 EXPERIMENTAL EVIDENCE

Neurophysiological data relating to the adaptive behavior of single or limited numbers of neurons will be reviewed to determine if the postulate of neuronal heterostasis is consistent with experimental results. Most of the evidence relating to large assemblies of neurons and whole nervous systems will be reviewed in Chapter 3.

The heterostatic model of the neuron offers the advantage of immediately suggesting a well-defined experimental test. What is required is the application of a depolarizing or hyperpolarizing bias to a neuron, while noting what long-term changes, if any, occur with respect to the neuron's average frequency of firing. Fortunately, such experiments have been performed and are reviewed next.

### 2.2.1  Neuronal and Cortical Polarization

A type of experiment that has been highly successful in producing effects resembling learning is that involving cortical polarization by means of small direct currents. Surface-positive polarization of the cortex has a depolarizing effect on neurons within the area of effect. According to the postulated neuronal model, if a neuron fires and depolarization follows, then the recently active excitatory synapses will increase in effectiveness. If hyperpolarization follows, the effectiveness of recently active inhibitory synapses will increase. We would, therefore, predict that surface-positive polarization of cortex should function as reward and surface-negative polarization should function as punishment. This prediction has been confirmed.

Rusinov (1953) discovered that surface-positive polarization of the rabbit's motor cortex resulted in limb responses for previously ineffective visual and auditory stimuli and, furthermore, the responses could be elicited for up to 30 minutes after cortical polarization ceased. Any stimulus that had been ineffective prior to polarization remained so afterward if it was not presented and responded to during polarization. The heterostatic model suggests that the continued response beyond the period of polarization resulted from increases in the transmittances of those excitatory synapses that were involved in producing the limb response during polarization. The polarization provides continuous positive reinforcement for these synapses. Rusinov's observations were later confirmed by Morrell (1961). The question remains as to why the apparent learning disappeared completely after 30 minutes. One possible explanation is that the experimental procedure did not produce a sufficient increase in the excitatory transmittances to prevent interference due to subsequent learning and changing patterns of neural activity. A more permanent form of learning is exhibited in the experiments described next.

Similar results were also obtained by Bindman, Lippold, and Redfearn (1964) using surface-positive and negative polarization. They state in their summary: "Surface-positive current enhances neuronal firing and increases the size of evoked potentials; surface-negative current has the opposite effect." Furthermore, "If current flow is prolonged for 5 to 10 minutes, a persistent aftereffect in the same direction is produced, lasting often without decrement, for at least 1 to 5 hours (p. 381)."

Bindman et al. (1964) also provided data with respect to highly localized neuronal behavioral changes involving at most about five neurons. In some of their experiments, instead of using surface polarization techniques, localized polarization was accomplished by passing a suitable current between a recording electrode (which doubled as a stimulator) and an indifferent electrode. In the rat cortex, tip-positive polarization that alone was insufficient to cause the neuron to fire nevertheless increased the average frequency of firing of neurons in the immediate vicinity of the electrode. Furthermore, the increased frequency resulting from tip-positive polarization was sustained by the neuron for up to 5 hours after stimulation ceased, if the duration of stimulation was at least 5 to 10 minutes. The heterostatic model predicts this result since the recording electrode was supplying a depolarizing bias that functioned as positive reinforcement each time the neuron fired. Active excitatory synapses were, therefore, undergoing increases in their transmittances during the period of stimulation. The model further predicts that the average frequency of firing should undergo a long-term *decrease* if tip-*negative* polarization, which causes hyperpolarization, is applied. Tip-negative polarization for 5 to 10 minutes, in fact, yielded a decreased average firing frequency that was maintained by the neuron after the polarizing electrode was turned off.

The changes in synaptic transmittances that were obtained in the above experiments by means of surface-positive and tip-positive polarization may also be obtained by stimulating subcortical facilitatory pathways (Bindman et al., 1964; Burns, 1968). Stimulation of a subcortical pathway for a period of time produced long-lasting increased cortical activity when the electrode stimulation forced the pathway involved to deliver a depolarizing bias, thereby causing some of the excitatory synaptic transmittances of recipient neurons to increase. This is an important observation because it suggests that physiological, as well as the above-described artificially induced, depolarization can have equivalent reinforcing effects on synaptic transmittances.

It is also relevant that cortical surface potential changes, similar to those artificially induced in the above-described experiments, have been observed to occur naturally during conditioning studies (Rowland and Goldstone, 1963; Walter et al., 1964). This is further evidence that cortical polarization simulates naturally occuring conditions of learning within the cortex.

Bures and Buresova (1970) have reviewed classical conditioning studies (see also Bures and Buresova, 1965, 1967; Gerbrandt et al., 1968) conducted "on nearly 250 neurons in the cerebral cortex, hippocampus, thalamus, and reticular formation of curarized unanesthetized rats. The classical conditioning paradigm was used throughout, the CS (acoustic or tactile stimulus) preceding and partly overlapping with the UCS (anodal or cathodal current applied through the recording extracellular micro-electrode)". They also report on single-cell conditioning studies utilizing the same US, but with a CS consisting of electrical stimulation of neurons in the close vicinity of the nerve cell. In this case, the CS was considered to be effective only when it resulted in impulses being delivered to the recorded cell. In both studies, about half of the neurons that exhibited a plastic reaction behaved in accordance with the heterostatic model and the experimental results reviewed above. However, the other half behaved in an opposite manner: a depolarizing US functioned as punishment and a hyperpolarizing US functioned as reward. These results suggest that either (a) more than one type of neuronal adaptive mechanism is to be found in the nervous system or (b) that the nonphysiological source of polarization has introduced uncontrolled variables producing the appearance of an inverse type of neuron. When polarization was provided by the more physiological means of subcortical stimulation (studies noted above) or in the production of a mirror focus (reviewed below), no "inverse" neurons were observed. Thus, we will continue to assume the existence of only the neuron type modeled earlier. If the inverse neuron does, in fact, occur, it will be necessary to revise the theory to include at least two types of adaptive neurons.

### 2.2.2  Epileptic Foci and the Mirror Focus

Along with neuronal and cortical polarization, the mirror focus appears to be one of the neurophysiological phenomena most capable of providing insights into the cellular mechanisms of learning (see review by Morrell, 1969). The procedure for inducing a mirror focus is a straightforward one. A primary epileptic focus, caused for instance by the localized freezing of cortical tissue, produces a secondary or "mirror" focus at a corresponding point in the opposite hemisphere. The effects of the primary focus reach the mirror focus via the corpus callosum. Initially, the secondary focus exhibits abnormal activity only in concert with the primary focus. The postulated neuronal model suggests that the depolarizing bias supplied by the primary focus should cause excitatory transmittances to increase at the mirror focus. Therefore, the mirror focus should eventually exhibit an abnormally high excitability independent of the primary focus. This is, indeed, what happens. After approximately one week, in the case of the rabbit, the primary focus may be removed and the mirror focus will continue independently. If the primary focus is removed before the end of the first week, an independent mirror focus is never established.

Morrell (1969) notes that a primary cortical focus may induce secondary epileptogenesis, not only in the opposite hemisphere, but also in subcortical structures such as thalamic (Wada and Cornelius, 1960) and limbic system nuclei (Guerrero-

Figueroa et al., 1964). Also, the primary focus may assume a subcortical location (Morrell, Proctor, and Prince, 1965; Proctor, Prince, and Morrell, 1966).

All of these observations are consistent with the assumption of a heterostatic neuron. Whenever a primary focus is established, it may be expected that it will induce abnormal neural assemblies in any area of the nervous system to which it projects a significant reinforcing bias. In fact, it is hypothesized that this is the mechanism by which epileptic seizures become progressively more extensive if unchecked by treatment. Specifically, the sequence of events in epilepsy is suggested to be the following:

1. A pathologic process causes an assembly of neurons to become hyperactive. Ward, Jasper, and Pope (1969) note that "seizure discharges may arise from such divergent reactions to injury as those associated with intracerebral traumatic lesions, chronic sepsis, infraction, neoplasis, and spontaneous, degenerative neuronal disease of many kinds."
2. The hyperactive assembly, once formed, imposes a depolarizing, hyperpolarizing, or mixed bias, depending upon the assembly's neural composition, on those neurons to which it sends its output.
3. Neurons receiving the bias undergo heterostatic adaptation, thus becoming hyper- or hypoactive assemblies themselves.
4. Formation of new assemblies continues until a stage is reached where either (a) the bias generated by the most recently formed assemblies is so weak or is distributed in such a diffuse manner as to be incapable of inducing the formation of further assemblies, or (b) the collection of assemblies forms a closed loop.

Viewing epilepsy as a progressive disease (Morrell and Baker, 1961) is supported not only by work on the mirror focus, but also more recently by the work of Goddard (1967). Goddard's observations provide further evidence that a depolarizing bias may induce the formation of an epileptic focus in a number of regions of the nervous system. Goddard implanted electrodes at various locations in the rat's brain and found that stimulation of only 50 $\mu$A for 1 minute per day, while posing no serious behavioral problems for the rat during the first few days, eventually produced convulsions. It appears that a permanent epileptic focus was established, because repetition of the stimulation, after being withheld for 3 months, yielded a convulsion once again. It is of interest that epileptic foci were established by Goddard in the amygdala after 15 days of stimulation, in the caudate putamen after 74 days, but not in the reticular formation even after 200 days of stimulation. Why epileptogenicity may vary as a function of the brain region is discussed in Chapter 3.

Some evidence relating to the spinal cord is relevant here. The spinal cord has been closely examined for synaptic changes associated with learning (Eccles, 1964, 1966), but these studies have not, in general, yielded evidence of long-term synaptic modifications. One exception concerns a phenomenon described in a review by Gurowitz (1969). After a unilateral cerebellar lesion, a rat experiences a postural asymmetry in the hind limbs. The asymmetry disappears if a midthoracic section is performed immediately following the lesion. However, if this section is delayed sufficiently, the asymmetry becomes permanent. Gurowitz states that "the asymmetry is considered to be the result of asymmetrical facilitatory stimulation via the descending spinal tracts." These observations suggest that the spinal cord is capable of learning when subjected to the influence of a depolarizing bias. This result, in combination with the evidence reviewed above, implies that most, if not all, neural tissue is capable of undergoing adaptation.

### 2.2.3 Modifiability of Synapses

While the evidence reviewed above indicates that synapses do undergo changes in their transmittances, or that some functional equivalent of this occurs, the cellular mechanism by which this is accomplished has, in the past, remained obscure. Whether new synapses are grown, old ones are lost, or existing ones are modified has been a matter for speculation. Variations in the amount of transmitter released or the extent of postsynaptic receptor sites are among the possible means that have been considered for achieving plasticity. Dendritic spines have appeared to be promising candidates for research on this question. Also, molecular mechanisms have been researched as a possible substrate for learning and memory. On the subject of synaptic variability, we will limit ourselves here to some speculation concerning which synapses are modifiable and whether the transmittances may undergo either increases or decreases, or both.

### 2.2.4 Experimental Tests

The machinery of the neuron that is available to implement heterostat-like adaptive mechanisms has been well discussed by Sutton and Barto (1979). Also, recent work by a number of investigators is providing an understanding of basic membrane biophysics and the biochemistry of the single neuron (e.g., see Woody, 1974 and 1977, or a review by Smith and Kreutzberg, 1976) such that it should now be possible to develop highly specific tests for heterostatic neuronal function. The experiments will involve, in effect, putting a single neuron in a Skinner box. Precise manipulation of transmitter (or second messenger) delivery to a neuron, both in terms of quantity and timing, perhaps using pressure microinjection techniques (Koike, Kandel, and Schwartz, 1974; Sakai, Swartz, Woody, 1979) would seem to open the way to rigorous testing of the hypothesized reinforcing effects of excitatory and inhibitory transmitters. In addition, recent clear demonstrations of plasticity obtained by Spinelli and Jensen (1979) offer alternative possibilities for linking the instrumental conditioning paradigm with adaptive changes in single neuron function.

## 2.3 VARIATIONS OF THE HETEROSTATIC MODEL

How many neuronal models will ultimately be required to explain adaptive brain function? In the present formulation of the heterostatic theory, we are assuming a single model, to see how far it will carry us. The experimental evidence might eventually require the adoption of multiple models. However, until this is demonstrated, we will continue to assume the most economical hypothesis consistent with the available evidence.

It might seem that at least two models will be required to explain adaptive neuronal function, one for excitatory and one for inhibitory neurons. Especially in a case like that of the cerebellum, which appears to work principally by inhibitory mechanisms (Eccles, Ito, and Szentagothai, 1967), it might seem that a second model would be required. However, the apparent dominance of inhibition in the cerebellum may only mean that cerebellar adaptation primarily involves inhibitory synapses and negative reinforcement, with the adaptive mechanism being like that proposed in Section 3.1. There seems to be no reason at this point to postulate different goals or adaptive mechanisms for excitatory and inhibitory plastic neurons, either for the case of the cerebellum or, more generally, for the whole nervous system.

Having said this, there are some variations of the heterostatic model that should, nevertheless, be considered. In the neuronal model that has been described, adaptation is accomplished with synaptic transmittances that undergo only increases in their absolute values. We will now consider some variations of the model that are obtained when other kinds of constraints are imposed on the variability of the transmittances. (In this discussion, we will always be referring to the absolute values of transmittances.) All of the models to be considered are equivalent in that they implement the basic heuristic already described which tends to maximize the amount of polarization experienced by the neuron.

Some of the constraints to be considered are those in which (a) synaptic transmittances increase only, (b) synaptic transmittances decrease only, (c) only excitatory synaptic transmittances vary, (d) only inhibitory synaptic transmittances vary, (e) only the transmittances associated with excitatory neurons vary, or (f) only the transmittances associated with inhibitory neurons vary. These possibilities, including some in combination, are shown in Table 1, which defines the types of heterostatic adaptive mechanisms to be commented on below.

### 2.3.1 Synaptic Transmittance Increases Only

A neuronal model in which synaptic transmittances can only increase (Type 1 adaptation) was described in Section 2.1. One

**TABLE 1.** Variations of the Heterostatic Model of the Neuron

| | | Direction of change of absolute value of transmittance (I = increase, D = decrease; where no symbol appears, synaptic transmittances is not modifiable). | | | |
|---|---|---|---|---|---|
| | | Excitatory neurons | | Inhibitory neurons | |
| Type of adaptive mechanism | Type of reinforcement[*] | Eligible excitatory synapses | Eligible inhibitory synapses | Eligible excitatory synapses | Eligible inhibitory synapses |
| 1 | P | I | | I | |
| | N | | I | | I |
| 2 | P | | D | | D |
| | N | D | | D | |
| 3 | P | I | | I | |
| | N | D | | D | |
| 4 | P | | D | | D |
| | N | | I | | I |
| 5 | P | I | | | |
| | N | | I | | |
| 6 | P | | | I | |
| | N | | | | I |
| 7 | P | | D | | |
| | N | D | | | |
| 8 | P | | | | D |
| | N | | | D | |
| 9 | P | I | | | |
| | N | D | | | |
| 10 | P | | | I | |
| | N | | | D | |
| 11 | P | | D | | |
| | N | | I | | |
| 12 | P | | | | D |
| | N | | | | I |

[*]This refers to the type of signals that impinge upon the neuron within the first few seconds after it fires. Depolarizing signal configurations constitute reward (positive); hyperpolarizing signal configurations constitute punishment (negative). P = positive, N = negative.

attractive feature of this kind of model is that a growth process could provide the basis for the transmittance changes. Furthermore, a model employing unidirectional transmittance changes might offer an explanation for the apparent loss of behavioral plasticity with increasing age. Bidirectional changes might be expected to provide a higher degree of flexibility for a nervous system, independent of how much experience had already been "read in." However, with a bidirectional system, the advantage of decreased rigidity might have an associated disadvantage: the increased ease of new learning might have to be purchased with an increased tendency to lose (overwrite) previously acquired information; that is, forgetting due to interference might be more of a problem with bidirectional transmittance changes.

## 2.3.2 Synaptic Transmittance Decreases Only

A neuronal model in which synaptic transmittances can only decrease (Type 2 adaptation) is the inverse of the case just described. If transmittances only decrease, adaptation could be realized by some kind of controlled decay process. Here, the transmittances would initially have to assume high values, whereas with Type 1 adaptation, the transmittances would initially assume low values.

## 2.3.3 Excitatory or Inhibitory Synapse Variations Only

We may consider a class of neuronal models in which transmittance modifications of only the excitatory (Type 3) or only the inhibitory (Type 4) synapses are permitted. In order to maintain the power of the adaptive process (that is, in order to still be able to reinforce positively *and* negatively), bidirectional transmittance changes must be utilized instead of the unidirectional changes employed with Type 1 and Type 2 adaptation.

It has been observed in some portions of the brain that excitatory synapses tend to be located on dendrites—especially on dendritic spines (Eccles, 1964)—whereas inhibitory synapses tend to be located on the soma or dentritic stump (Andersen, Eccles, Lyning, 1963; Anderson, Eccles, and Voorhoeve, 1963; Blackstad and Flood, 1963). If the mechanism of transmittance variability is located only within the dendrites—for example, if it is associated with the dendritic spines—then Type 3 adaptation may be a relevant model because it leaves inhibitory synaptic transmittances fixed. But then, as noted above, the modifiable transmittances must be capable of changing in both directions. Bidirectional changes might mean that the part of the neuron corresponding to the transmittance-modifying mechanism would have to be more complex than in the case of Type 1 or Type 2 adaptation.

Type 4 adaptation might be the appropriate model of the neuronal adaptive process if it should turn out that only axosomatic synaptic transmittances are modifiable.

### 2.3.4 Adaptation in Only Excitatory or Inhibitory Neurons

The latter eight types of adaptive mechanisms shown in Table 1 (Types 5-12) represent variations of the first four types. In these eight models, we examine several ways of obtaining adaptive processes that possess essentially all of the power of the first four types, but require that fewer of the synapses be modifiable. The power of these eight types of adaptive mechanisms is reduced from that of the first four types only to the extent that fewer modifiable synapses are available to store the information of learning and memory. But this is a minor consideration. The important point is that the fundamental nature of the adaptive mechanism is unchanged with any of the 12 models shown in Table 1. Types 5 through 12 differ from Types 1 through 4 in that the modifiable transmittances are restricted to either the excitatory or inhibitory neurons, depending on the model. The models in which only the inhibitory neurons are adaptive might be relevant for the cerebellum where, as noted earlier, it has been observed that inhibition dominates information processing.

In the chapters that follow, Type 1 adaptation will be assumed for the purpose of discussion. However, none of the arguments presented would be substantially altered if one of the other models were adopted.

# Chapter 3
# **psychology**

In this chapter, the assumption of a heterostatic neuron provides the basis for speculation concerning the neurophysiological mechanisms that underlie psychological phenomena. The question of the mind-body relationship is taken up and consideration is given to the global organization of the brain.

## 3.1 LEARNING

### 3.1.1 Habituation

Nervous systems become habituated to redundant stimuli while continuing to respond to novel and significant inputs. It is proposed that two types of localized neural circuitry are important in understanding this behavior. These two circuit types are feed-forward and recurrent inhibition, both of which, Eccles (1969a) has noted, are found throughout the central nervous sytem. Feed-forward inhibition makes it probable that when a neuron fires, some inhibitory synapses will have been active. This insures that recently active inhibitory synapses will generally be available to undergo increases in their transmittances should hyperpolarization follow impulse generation. Recurrent inhibition guarantees that hyperpolarization will follow impulse generation, thus causing the inhibitory synapses associated with the original stimulus to become increasingly effective, unless sufficient facilitation arrives to counter the local inhibitory feedback. Evidence of the increasing effectiveness of inhibitory synapses during habituation has been obtained by Holmgren and Frenk (1961) in their study of the pleural ganglion of the snail. It can be seen that extensive feed-forward and recurrent inhibition provides neurons with the means for what is, in effect, self-habituation. Only the intervention of positive reinforcement (excitation) sufficient to counteract the local recurrent inhibition can save a stimulus from the neural judgment of irrelevance.

That the frontal cortex can markedly accelerate habituation is supported by much research (see review by Griffin, 1970). In the context of the present theory, this suggests that the process of encephalization has resulted in the frontal cortex becoming a primary source of inhibition to be utilized during the habituation process. It may be that frontal lobe inhibition can be generated in much the same manner as recurrent inhibition, that is, as an inhibitory feedback response to neuronal firing, but covering much greater distances. This type of inhibition may be termed *extended recurrent inhibition* to distinguish it from *local recurrent inhibition* as discussed by Eccles (1969a).

A primary source of the counteracting facilitation, when habituation is avoided, is likely to be the limbic system and the hypothalamus (henceforth collectively designated as the LSH). It is postulated that the LSH, using genetically specified mechanisms, identifies stimuli relevant to the animal's needs (these are the unconditioned stimuli) and then delivers facilitation to many parts of the brain. Actually, this postulated LSH action applies only to appetitive unconditioned stimuli. Defensive unconditioned stimuli will be discussed later, along with a more detailed discussion of the LSH's reinforcement centers.

It is now possible to understand what happens when a novel stimulus (a potential conditioned stimulus) is processed by the reticular formation (RF), for example. First, it has been noted that the RF is always aroused by a novel stimulus, which indicates that excitatory synapses of excitatory RF neurons dominate over inhibitory synapses, at least initially. However, after the RF receives the stimulus, if the LSH is not aroused within a few seconds (by the arrival of an unconditioned stimulus) and, therefore, the LSH does not supply facilitation to the RF, then frontal lobe inhibition, arising out of the RF's initial response, will cause active RF neurons to be punished; that is, hyperpolarization will follow impulse generation and recently active inhibitory synapses of the RF will undergo increases in their transmittances. With repetitive presentations of the stimulus, these inhibitory transmittances will continue to increase until the neurons of the RF no longer respond. In a similar fashion, habituation may occur elsewhere, such as in the cortex, where local or extended recurrent inhibition, or both, may be active.

### 3.1.2 Dishabituation

Responses to previously habituated stimuli, that is, dishabituation, results when (a) the habituated stimulus is withheld for a period of time, (b) a novel stimulus is presented prior to the habituated stimulus, or (c) the habituated stimulus is presented simultaneously with another stimulus. In all of these cases, dishabituation is hypothesized to be due to the nervous system assuming a significantly different state of activity when the habituated stimulus is presented again so that a new set of synapses will undergo increases in their transmittances and habituation will be established once more. In this way, inhibition relative to a particular stimulus becomes even more extensive and it, therefore, becomes progressively more difficult to dishabituate a stimulus following repeated habituation. The suggestion of Spencer, Thompson, and Neilson, (1969a, 1969b) that a dishabituating stimulus has a generalized facilitatory effect further explains how increased inhibitory transmittances can be overridden during dishabituation.

Habituation is often highly specific to the stimulus presented. Slight changes in the stimulus can cause the animal to respond again. This is reasonable because the increased inhibitory transmittances mediating habituation will be of such a magnitude as to only minimally inhibit the neurons involved. Minimal inhibition occurs because, as postulated in Chapter 2, a neuron must fire if synaptic modifications are to follow. For this reason, as soon as the inhibitory transmittances increase just enough to terminate the neuronal response, the transmittances cannot increase further. In this situation, it can be seen that inhibition will have only a very small edge over excitation. Therefore, when even a small number of the synapses with increased inhibitory transmittances are not utilized, such as in the case of a slightly different stimulus, the animal once again may respond. The hypothesis that habituation involves minimal inhibition also explains why dishabituation can occur so easily.

It should be noted that more than minimal inhibition could develop during habituation if stimulus presentations continued beyond the zero response level. In this case, some neurons may still be responding (although without causing any observable behavioral effect) and these neurons will themselves become habituated. Under such circumstances, habituation could become more extensive. In this case, one might expect habituated "stimulus generalization," that is, lack of response to a broad class of stimuli that resembles the original stimulus but are not identical to it. Both habituation beyond the zero response level and habituated stimulus generalization have been observed experimentally and are discussed in a review by Thompson and Spencer (1966).

The habituation mechanism discussed above is supported by the observation that inhibitory neurons of the cerebrum, when they are induced to fire, continue to do so for about 200 to 500 ms (Eccles, 1966). This period resembles the optimal CS-US interval of conditioning studies, indicating that the cerebral inhibitory neuron is well suited for its role as a generator of inhibitory reinforcement. On the other hand, Eccles notes that inhibitory neurons in the spinal cord are not capable of this kind of long-term firing; instead, a single volley lasts for no more than 20 ms. Also, the amplitude of the spinal IPSP is, at most, one-tenth of that for cerebral inhibitory neurons. Since reinforcing signals do not appear to have their maximal effect on a neuron until approximately 400 ms have elapsed after impulse generation, one would expect habituation to proceed slowly, if at all, in the spinal cord. This is consistent with observation. For example, cervical transection of the spinal cord of a kitten, performed to eliminate the influence of higher centers, yields an animal that requires 2 weeks of training before habituation of the withdrawal reflex will occur (Meldrum, 1966). In the intact animal, habituation to a stimulus is accomplished within a few trials.

Since the evidence suggests that there are two basic types of inhibitory neurons, it would be of interest to know exactly how they are distributed throughout the CNS. This question assumes new significance because the present theory suggests that one of the two types is especially well suited for use in adaptive circuits. Eccles (1969a) has reviewed evidence suggesting that inhibitory neurons having a short-duration IPSP are restricted to the spinal cord, while inhibitory neurons at suprasegmental levels are of the long-duration IPSP type. This distribution has been deduced on the basis of observations of the depressant action of strychnine, which affects only inhibitory neurons having short-duration IPSP's. The observed distribution is interesting because it shows that the midbrain is the lowest level at which we find inhibitory neurons that are well suited for the purpose of generating extended recurrent inhibitory reinforcement. Penfield has reviewed evidence suggesting that the midbrain and thalamic regions of the brain stem are of critical importance for the maintenance of conscious awareness. Penfield (1969) notes that "compression or injury in this region . . . extinguishes awareness and is followed by amnesia (p. 800)." Thus, adaptive circuits appropriate to such learning phenomena as rapid habituation seem to appear at just that level in the CNS which may also serve as the seat of consciousness.

Habituation below the midbrain may be accomplished by an entirely different mechanism than that employed at or above the midbrain. This suggestion is supported by a study of the bulbar reticular formation (Segundo, Takenaka, and Encabo, 1967) in which the investigators concluded that habituation occurred because "interneuronal pools have junctions whose activation is followed by prolonged subnormality [of the presynaptic terminal]." Such a mechanism appears to resemble those found by Kandel (1974) and others in simple nervous systems such as aplysia.

### 3.1.3  Classical Conditioning

In this discussion of Pavlovian conditioning and that which follows on operant conditioning, only appetitive reflexes will be considered. Defensive reflexes will be considered later, after the role of pain in nervous systems has been analyzed.

The proposed neuronal model is consistent with the observation that no conditioning occurs with simultaneous presentation of the CS and US. The optimal CS-US interval, as already noted, is approximately 400 ms, with the US becoming completely ineffective if the interval exceeds a few seconds (see review by Russell, 1966).

In the following discussion, the sets of neurons that fire in response to the presentation of a CS or US will be denoted by {CS} and {US}, respectively. The neuronal model predicts that when these sets are sequentially active within a few seconds of one another, those neurons belonging to the intersection, {CS} $\wedge$ {US}, will be positively reinforced. That is to say, excitatory synapses of the neurons belonging to the intersection will undergo increases in their transmittances if these synapses were activated by the CS but not activated (and thus zero set) by the US. The LSH's response to the US may also be a source of positive reinforcement for neurons in {CS}. The effect of both kinds of reinforcement during conditioning will be to cause the sets {CS} and {CS} $\wedge$ {US} to increase in size and average frequency of firing. As these increases occur for the set, {CS} $\wedge$ {US}, one would expect an increasing resemblance between the CR and the UR, as indeed happens. However, because the intersection set, {CS} $\wedge$ {US}, will, in general, contain only a fraction of the neurons in {US}, the CR is a fractional component of the UR (Konorski, 1948); that is, the CR and UR do not become identical as was once thought.

Recently, Sutton and Barto (1979) have proposed a classical conditioning model derived from the heterostat (Klopf, 1972). Combining expectation and prediction mechanisms proposed by Sutton (1978a) with aspects of the heterostatic adaptive mechanism we have been discussing here, Sutton and Barto have demonstrated that the resulting adaptive element (1) "learns to increase its response rate in anticipation of increased stimulation, producing a CR before the occurrence of the UCS," (2) "is in strong agreement with the behavioral data regarding the effects of stimulus context," (3) "becomes sensitive to the most reliable, non-redundant and earliest predictors of reinforcement" and (4) "solves many of the stability and saturation problems encountered in network simulations." Thus, a heterostat-like model appears to be highly successful in capturing those aspects of classical conditioning that have also been modeled well by such investigators as Rescorla and Wagner (1972) and, beyond that, captures many of the temporal aspects of classical conditioning faithfully.

### 3.1.4  Operant Conditioning

In the following discussion, CS, CR, US, and UR refer to instrumental stimuli and responses. The sets, {CS} and {US}, are defined as in the case of classical conditioning.

Whenever a CS-CR sequence occurs, a US that follows within a few seconds causes the LSH (according to our earlier hypothesis) to supply positive reinforcement to {CS}, thereby causing the active excitatory synapses of {CS} to undergo increases in their transmittances. As these transmittances continue to increase with further conditioning, the CR follows the CS with increasing reliability. Where the CR occurs spontaneously (i.e., is not preceded by the CS nor followed by the US), habituation eventually eliminates the response because there is no US to arouse the LSH and, therefore, no positively reinforcing facilitation.

With continued repetition of the CS-CR sequence and with an appetitive US, there is nothing to prevent excitatory synapses from continuing to increase far beyond the minimal level required to produce the conditioned response. Thus, for the same reason that we predicted that habituation would generalize, we can predict that conditioned stimuli should also generalize, since the large transmittance values will make it unnecessary that every excitatory synapse involved in the response to the original stimulus be active in order to obtain the same kind of response to a modified stimulus. This type of generalization does occur; a variety of stimuli similar to the CS can evoke the CR (see review by Russell, 1966).

In this and the previous section, it has been demonstrated that the heterostatic neuronal model offers a single adaptive mechanism as an explanation for both classical and operant conditioning. Sutton (1978b) has reached a similar conclusion in an analysis of the implications of heterostatic adaptation for learning phenomena.

### 3.1.5  Extinction

When a classical or operant CS ceases to be reinforced, extinction of the response eventually occurs. It is proposed that the mechanism involved is the same as for habituation. It is suggested, therefore, that local and extended recurrent inhibition are involved. An identity of the underlying mechanisms of habituation and extinction has been considered by others (Sharpless, 1964; Thompson and Spencer, 1966). Furthermore, Kling and Stevenson (1970) note that "The theories of extinction cited most often have postulated some process of inhibition." They cite Pavlov's (1927) and Hull's (1943) theories as examples.

The fact that extinction proceeds more slowly and erratically than habituation can be understood if one considers that the CS not only becomes associated with the CR, but may also become associated with the US. That is, the CS becomes conditioned to activate not only the CR, but also a portion of the set {US}, and, in this way, the CR becomes partially self-reinforcing. Thus, when the US is no longer presented, the set {US} may still be partially active, following the occurrence of the CS-CR sequence. It is concluded that this partial acitivity of the set, {US}, causes the extinction of the CS-CR association to proceed more slowly and erratically than the normal process of habituation.

This ability of a CS to become associated with a US, as well as with a CR, thereby providing the CS with a dual role, is, perhaps, what permits long behavioral chains to develop, such as in the running of a maze. In such a chain, leading ultimately to a "true" US, an intermediate stimulus comes to serve as a CS with respect to the next response and as a US with respect to the preceding response.

The ability of an extinguished response to reappear after only a very small amount of renewed conditioning is reasonable, due to the fact that only minimal inhibition would be expected to develop during the extinction process. As in the case of habituation, minimal inhibition occurs because the inhibitory transmittances stop increasing immediately upon cessation of the response. Thus, only small increases in excitatory transmittances will be necessary for the previously extinguished response to appear again.

## 3.2 THE MIND-BODY PROBLEM

Having provided experimental support for the heterostatic neuronal model at both the neurophysiological and psychological levels, we can now consider, in a more complete fashion, what the heterostatic model implies for the global organization of the brain. It will be useful first to take up the issue of the mind-body problem.

Four recent and thoroughgoing reviews are especially relevant to this section and, more generally, to the present monograph. Readers who have a deep interest in the mind-body problem will want to be familiar with Thatcher and John's (1977) *Foundations of Cognitive Processes*, Uttal's (1978) *The Psychobiology of Mind*, Gazzaniga and LeDoux's (1978) *The Integrated Mind*, and Luria's (1978) paper, *The Human Brain and Conscious Activity*.

### 3.2.1 Animals Are Heterostats

If the constituent elements of a given system seek a common goal, it is plausible that the total system will seek the same goal. Thus, we might expect that nervous systems consisting of heterostatic neurons would seek as their overall goal to obtain depolarizing experiences and to avoid hyperpolarizing experiences. More precisely, it is suggested that such nervous systems tend to maximize the average amount of neuronal polarization experienced. Thus, it is postulated that advanced organisms are heterostats.

### 3.2.2 An Identity Theory

Because it is generally observed, or readily interpreted, that humans and, by implication, other advanced animals seek to obtain pleasure and to avoid pain, it was hypothesized earlier that pleasure and pain are the psychological counterparts of the physicalistic concepts of depolarization and hyperpolarization, respectively. This basis for a solution of the mind-body problem is proposed as an identity theory (Feigl, 1958, 1960; Pepper, 1960; Globus, 1976) of the $\Phi - \Psi$ (physiological-psychological) relationship.

The suggestion is that pleasure and pain, in the form of single neurons undergoing depolarization or hyperpolarization respectively, constitute the two fundamental "psychic atoms" out of which all of our more complex mental states are constructed. ("Psychic" and "mental" are synonymous in this discussion.) Each neuron may be thought of as generating a psychic field during polarization, this field corresponding to some as yet unidentified aspects of the polarization process. We may consider that there are *d-fields* and *h-fields*, resulting from depolarization and hyperpolarization, respectively.

It is further suggested that the psychic fields of individual neurons combine to form more complex psychic fields and thus arises the entity termed "mind." If this proposal seems far-fetched, consider that if the concept of mind is ever to be related to physical processes, the processes will have to be located in individual neurons and then "integrated" to form the more complex entity we term conscious awareness. If we wish to explain the phenomenon of consciousness without integrating primitive psychic fields to obtain more complex fields, our only alternative would seem to be that of associating our conscious-ness with processes *in a single neuron*. This hypothesis seems less plausible than that requiring the integration of multiple primitive fields.

A proposal by Pribram (1966, 1971) is related to the hypothesis suggested here. In summarizing his proposal, Pribram (1976) states that "the essential mechanism involved in the production of awareness is the pattern of local graded potential changes, the depolarizations and hyperpolarizations which occur at synaptic junctions and in dendritic networks." In the present theory, we are accepting the idea of an identity between neuronal potential changes and mental phenomena and then going further to associate depolarization specifically with pleasure and hyperpolarization specifically with pain.

### 3.2.3 Defining Consciousness

"Consciousness" seems like a difficult term to define. However, the difficulties that are encountered are often due to confusion regarding the mind-body problem. Actually, consciousness can be defined in a straightforward way that is consistent with many aspects of general usage of the term. A conscious system may be defined as one that contains a model of itself, its environment, and the relationship of itself to its environment. Consciousness, then, is the experience of being a model of the self, the environment, and the relationship of the two. Consciousness defined in this way is an emergent property of brains, a property that is acquired as experience and learning provide increasing information with which to define the self, the environment, and their relationship. In accordance with this definition, newborn infants are conscious only to a slight degree. We can speak of degrees of consciousness just as we can speak of degrees of accuracy of an internal model.

Defining consciousness in this way removes some of the mystery that has, at times, unnecessarily shrouded this subject. There has been a tendency in the past to confuse simple responsiveness in living systems with consciousness, although the two are fundamentally different. Consciousness has also been associated with the idea of simply having a "mental" existence, that is, having such experiences as those of pleasure and pain in their elementary or complex forms. However, past and current speculation on the mind-body problem suggests that mental phenomena such as pleasure and pain may be as pervasive within the universe as electromagnetic fields or matter itself (e.g., see Globus, 1976; Thatcher and John, 1977). If such is the case, our definition of consciousness must be narrowed if the term is to remain useful. The definition proposed here is an attempt to accomplish this, as well as to provide a definition that is consistent with the implications of adaptive network research (e.g., see Somerhoff, 1974) and artificial intelligence research (e.g., see Minsky, 1969a).

### 3.2.4 Localization of Consciousness

What is the substrate of consciousness? Currently, many investigators favor a view like that advocated by Sperry (1975):

[A] view that reached a peak in the 1950's (Delafresnaye, 1954) had consciousness centered in brainstem reticular and centrencephalic mechanisms. The contention was that a person really lives, so far as conscious feeling and experience are concerned, in these deep mesencephalic centers. The neocortex came to be regarded as a relatively recent and superficial adjunct for enhancing and elaborating the basic qualities of conscious experience already evolved in the mesencephalon. Interpretations along these lines had to be largely abandoned in the face of our new findings on brain bisection in which surgical separation of the cerebral hemispheres alone, leaving the brainstem intact, proved sufficient to divide most of the higher psychological functions in cats and primates. (p. 429)

There is an alternative to Sperry's interpretation, an alternative that returns us to the 1950s view that Sperry has rejected. Let us consider the following question. When consciousness appears to be split after disconnecting the cerebral hemispheres, is that because consciousness resides in those hemispheres, as Sperry suggests, or is it because consciousness resides in the reticular formation that is intimately tied to the two hemispheres? There are a number of reasons for considering the reticular formation as a candidate location for consciousness. The reticular formation occupies a strategic anatomical location providing access to information from most parts of the nervous system. The reticular formation, at the medullary, midbrain, and thalamic levels, has been hypothesized to serve as the command and control center for the brain (Kilmer, McCulloch, and Blum, 1967, 1969; see also Kilmer, 1975). It has been suggested that the RF commits us at any given moment to one of approximately two dozen possible gross modes of behavior such as running, fighting, mating, eating, or sleeping. As noted earlier, evidence reviewed by Penfield (1969) is consistent with the localization of conscious processes within the mesencephalon and diencephalon, and, in fact, Penfield (1975) adopted such a hypothesis (see also important reviews by Fessard, 1954; John, 1976). We have also reviewed evidence that showed that long-duration IPSP neurons, which appear to be well suited as adaptive circuit elements, occur at the level of the midbrain and above, but not below. It is on the basis of these considerations that it is hypothesized that the midbrain and thalamic reticular formation (MTRF) is the seat of the mental experiences of which we are aware. An alternative hypothesis is that the seat of consciousness is restricted to the thalamic reticular formation. Evidence reviewed by Weil (1974) suggests this possibility.

If, indeed, the reticular formation is the seat of consciousness, then it appears that the RF speaks for us via the cortical speech center. The other brain structures are then mute, having to be content with a lesser understanding of affairs going on about them and with only an indirect influence on the speech process that is fundamental to advanced forms of consciousness. The other brain structures probably experience pleasure and pain but, apparently, the nature of psychic fields is such that those fields associated with other brain structures do not significantly interact with the psychic field of the MTRF. Thus, we are no more aware of the psychic field associated with our own cortex, for example, than we are of the psychic field associated with someone else's cortex.

In considering the localization of consciousness, one line of evidence should be noted because it has been interpreted as ruling out the reticular formation as a candidate site. Thatcher and John (1977) summarize the evidence as follows:

> ... the conclusion that the reticular formation was the site where conscious processes were localized or that it was essential for consciousness, a view to which many were and still are inclined, was invalidated by such studies as those of Adametz (1959) and Chow (1961), showing that if the reticular formation was damaged bilaterally with lesions ... inflicted in several stages, no interference with consciousness or arousal was observed. Nonetheless, although the reticular formation may not be essential for consciousness, it seems to play an important role in the mediation of conscious processes in the intact brain. (p. 290)

An alternative interpretation of these ablation studies is that serial lesions provide time for adaptation and thereby for transfer of function to surrounding neural tissue. Adametz's and Chow's results do not rule out the possibility that the function of consciousness originally resided, at least in part, at the lesioned site.

Historically, the tendency to favor the cerebral cortex as the seat of consciousness was due to the belief that consciousness was largely or exclusively a property of humans. It directly followed that the human's quantitatively distinctive cortex should be the seat of that consciousness. Also, mediating against the brain stem as the seat of consciousness is the inclination to think that if a brain structure is phylogenetically old, its function must be primitive. Thus, the brain stem has sometimes been referred to as part of the "reptilian brain" (MacLean, 1962, 1964).

On the other hand, supporting the hypothesis that the MTRF is the seat of consciousness are observations associated with, in fact, the split-brain phenomenon. A "split-brain" results from partial disconnection of the cerebral hemispheres by sectioning of the corpus callosum and the anterior commissure. The results of this surgical procedure, especially in humans, have appeared remarkable to researchers. Gazzaniga (1972) has said, "In many ways, the split-brain phenomenon is as startling and basically mysterious today as when R. E. Myers and R. W. Sperry first discovered it in animals in the early fifties (p. 311)." The mysteries Gazzaniga (1972) refers to revolve around such conclusions as the following: "It would seem fair to say that we now know that the physical substrate of conscious experience exists in duplicate in the human brain (p. 317)." Also, "We know beyond a shadow of a doubt that it is [the corpus callosum] which relates the psychological, conscious experiences of one hemisphere to the other (p. 316)." If one accepts these conclusions, it is, indeed, surprising that sectioning of the corpus callosum in humans produces, as Gazzaniga (1967) has noted, "no noticeable change in the patients' temperament, personality or general intelligence (p. 24)." However, such unexpected results become easier to understand if one adopts the hypothesis that the MTRF is the seat of consciousness, in which case, the integrity of the physical substrate of the mind is preserved in split-brains.

The hypothesized role of the MTRF as the command and control center and seat of consciousness can be better appreciated by comparing the global organization of the human brain with that of the digital computer. Brain-computer comparisons have been very much overdone in recent years so it needs to be emphasized that, in most respects, brains and computers are fundamentally different. However, it is instructive to compare aspects of the global organizations of these two kinds of systems.

In the case of the digital computer, decision making and computing occurs in the central processing unit (CPU). But, while the CPU is the heart of the system, it may be only a small fraction of the total system in terms of its size. As computers grow larger and more powerful, most of the growth is due to the addition of extensive memories and I/O devices that surround the CPU. In the evolution of nervous systems, a similar global architecture appears to have emerged. As animals more advanced than the reptile evolved, it is hypothesized that the reticular formation (corresponding to the digital computer's CPU) has continued to serve as the command and control center and the seat of consciousness. The evolution of the LSH represented the addition of a relatively primitive form of memory, I/O capability and auxiliary processor. This was followed by the evolution of a truly sophisticated memory, I/O capability and extensive auxiliary processor in the form of the cerebral hemispheres. In this way, the MTRF has acquired the "peripheral equipment" that permits it to function, in the case of the human, as a truly powerful conscious command and control center.

With this view of the global organization of the brain, the roles of the corpus callosum and the speech center, as observed in human split-brain phenomena, can be better understood. If the elaborate internal model that is consciousness is dynamically maintained in the reticular formation and, further, if the model is maintained by means of vast numbers of feedback loops between the RF and the neocortex (these loops being an aspect of the function of the so-called reticular activating system), then, because of the close coupling of the cerebral hemispheres with the reticular formation, we would expect the very kinds of effects obtained in split-brain studies. For example, it would appear that the corpus callosum is needed to "set up" the speech center so that when the MTRF directs it to do so, the speech center can speak for the contents of the minor hemisphere. Eye movement and the use of both hands can make the corpus callosum largely redundant, but not completely so, as careful experimentation has demonstrated (see reviews by Gazzaniga, 1967, 1972). An indication of the redundance of the corpus callosum, at least from a gross perspective, is the fact that people who never developed this structure (for congenital reasons) are not behaviorally distinguishable from people with a normal brain structure (Ettlinger, et al., 1974).

If, at times, the corpus callosum seems redundant, so, too, do the cerebral hemispheres. The tendency, especially in the popular press in recent years, to emphasize right brain-left brain differences has been countered by Gazzaniga and LeDoux (1978) who note substantial functional similarities between the two hemispheres. Also, in this regard, a discussion by Puccetti (1973) is interesting:

> Consider . . . in the monumental study by Bogen (1969), evidence cited of 185 cases involving gross ablations or even complete hemispherectomy where there remained a 'person,' no matter which hemisphere was gone. Now if the person were unitary despite the duality of mind Bogen postulates, it ought to be the case that only half the original person has survived. Yet over and over again clinical reports suggest that essentially the same personality, character traits and long term memory traces persist postoperatively. The only way I can see to explain this is to say the same 'person' did not survive hemispherectomy at all. Because this former 'person' was never a unitary person to begin with. He or she was a compound of two persons who functioned in concert by transcommissural exchange. What has survived is one of two *very similar* persons with roughly parallel memory traces, nearly synchronous emotional states, perceptual experiences, and so on, but differential processing functions. (p. 352)

Of course, an alternative to Puccetti's interpretation is that there is only one "person" to begin with and that this "person" resides in the MTRF, receiving support from massive "auxiliary processors" in the form of the substantially redundant cerebral hemispheres. This would seem to be a simpler explanation of the fact that, in cases of partial or complete hemispherectomy, as Puccetti (1973) notes, essentially the same personality, character traits, and long term memory traces persist postoperatively.

With respect to language-dependent information processing, split-brain data (Sperry, 1966; Gazzaniga, 1970) indicate that the integration of information from the left and right sides of the body is accomplished at the cortical level, that is, above the level of the MTRF. When the MTRF is aware of events associated with the left side of the body, as demonstrated through speech or writing, it would appear that the MTRF obtains this awareness by interrogating the left dominant hemisphere which, in turn, receives reports from the right hemisphere. This argument is based on the fact that sectioning of the corpus callosum, the anterior and hippocampal commissures, and the massa intermedia (done for the purpose of controlling severe epileptic seizures), renders a person unable to communicate information via speech or writing if the information is available only to the left side of the body or to the left half of the visual field. Furthermore, the right side of the body is no longer able to act on the basis of information available only to the left side. All of this evidence points to a very high degree of coupling between the dominant hemisphere and that portion of the RF which is hypothesized to be the seat of conscious awareness. The alternative interpretation is that the evidence is pointing directly to the localization of consciousness in the cerebral hemispheres. The above discussion, however, is intended to show that the evidence does not require this interpretation. Considering all of the available evidence, it seems most likely that evolution has not led to the encephalization of the command and control function that we know as consciousness.

An observation relating to sensory deprivation phenomena is relevant while considering the role of the MTRF as a command and control center. Viewing the MTRF as a central processing unit that is continually driven by its vast array of inputs makes it clear why the effects of sensory deprivation are generally deleterious. MTRF inputs constitute, collectively, the forcing function that drives the MTRF through successive states, sometimes referred to as the "stream of consciousness." Sensory deprivation, in drastically altering the forcing function, presents the MTRF with a situation where its synaptic transmittances are inappropriate. The result is a command and control center that, in extreme circumstances, goes berserk.

### 3.2.5 Quantitative Aspects of Mental Phenomena

The intensity with which we experience pleasure or pain is hypothesized to be approximately proportional to the absolute difference between the number of MTRF neurons undergoing depolarization, denoted by $Q(D)$, and the number undergoing hyperpolarization, denoted by $Q(H)$. Therefore, positive and negative differences for the quantity

$$\Delta(t) = Q_t(D) - Q_t(H) \tag{18}$$

correspond to pleasurable and painful mental states, respectively. The terms pleasure and pain are used in a most general sense here, denoting all psychic states as either agreeable or disagreeable.

The kind of pleasure or pain experienced (e.g., love, hatred, joy, or grief) is hypothesized to depend on the particular configuration of depolarizing and hyperpolarizing events occurring within the MTRF at a given moment. To make this notion explicit, we may define an *MTRF state vector*, $\overline{\text{MTRF}}$, which has one component for each neuron in the midbrain and thalamic reticular formation. Each component will always assume one of three values representing the momentary state of the corresponding neuron. Thus, the MTRF state vector

$$\overline{\text{MTRF}}(t) = (R, D, D, H, \dots) \tag{19}$$

indicates that at time, $t$, neuron 1 is in the resting state $(R)$, neurons 2 and 3 are undergoing depolarization $(D)$, and neuron 4 is undergoing hyperpolarization $(H)$. The dimensionality of the state vector is estimated to be that of a $10^9$-tuple since the total number of neurons for humans is estimated to be $10^{12}$ and the RF of higher vertebrates has been estimated to constitute about 1/1000 (Kilmer, McCulloch, and Blum, 1967) of the CNS.

In accordance with the assumptions noted above, it is expected that the set of all possible mental states maps into the set of all possible MTRF state vectors. The state vector, $\overline{\text{MTRF}}$, specifies the particular mental state of the organism, that is, the *kind* of pleasure or pain being experienced. The *delta value*, as defined by Eq. (18), measures the degree of pleasure or pain experienced.

Since there are an extremely large number $(3^{10^9})$ of possible MTRF state vectors, there is a similarly large number of possible mental states. However, it appears to be the case with the human brain that the range of mental states is encompassed within the three major categories of feeling tone, sensation, and ideation. It is hypothesized that these three broad classifications correspond to states where the LSH, sensory cortex, and nonsensory-nonmotor cortex, respectively, supply the principal inputs driving the MTRF. Pratt (1937) observed that "Feeling tone is notably different from sensation and ideation. It is less objective; it is relatively independent of external objects and peripheral stimulation (p. 291)." When one considers the higher information content that would seem to be involved with sensation and ideation, it appears reasonable that only the mental experience corresponding to feeling tone might be compatible with high delta values.

When inputs from the LSH are the primary ones driving the MTRF, it is expected that a large portion of the MTRF neurons will be simultaneously either excited or inhibited, depending on whether the LSH is delivering excitatory or inhibitory reinforcement. In these circumstances, we refer to the experience as one of emotion; the MTRF is being driven by what may amount to high amplitude, low resolution inputs. When MTRF inputs from the sensory cortex predominate, we report the experience of sensations and when the nonsensory-nonmotor cortex predominates, we report the experience of memories or ideas. It is anticipated that the mix of excited and inhibited neurons within the MTRF is more nearly balanced in the case of sensations, memories, or ideas than when LSH inputs are "washing over" this structure. If this is so, then cortical inputs to the MTRF represent low amplitude, high resolution signals.

### 3.2.6 The $\Phi$ of $\Phi - \Psi$

If our speculation thus far on the mind-body problem bears some useful resemblance to the true state of affairs, what then might be the observable physical variables that are identical with the psychic variables? Speculation along three lines seems promising.

First, it would appear that we need to look for a field phenomenon. Otherwise, one has to integrate over something as discrete as individual neurons and come up with something possessing the apparent unity of the mind. As Sherrington (1941) observed, "Matter and energy seem granular in structure . . . but not so mind." If we do require a field, a natural candidate for the role is, of course, the electromagnetic field. Can it be that elementary pleasure and pain are one and the same, respectively, as the collapsing and expanding electromagnetic fields that arise during the neuronal polarization process? Is the mind identical with the electromagnetic field generated collectively by MTRF neurons? [Thatcher and John (1977) have examined a related possibility that they term the "hyperneuron."]

An alternative lies in the wave properties of matter itself. When we look inside a head, what we see is "physiological tissue." But, of course, what we *see* in the head is not what is there. We see physiological tissue, but physiological tissue is a *representation* (in our own heads) of what is there; it is not the thing, itself. If we want to know the thing itself, we turn to the physicist for a characterization of matter and energy. And what does the physicist say? That the behavior of matter and energy are described perfectly in quantum theoretic terms, i.e., strictly in terms of *wave* equations. Thus, in more objective terms, what we find inside the head appear to be wave phenomena! Could not these wave phenomena (or some portion of them) be one and the same thing as consciousness? In this view, "mental" descriptions result when we describe consciousness from the inside and "physical" descriptions result when we describe consciousness from the outside. We have two descriptions of a single thing. Such an identity theory appears to offer the simplest and most plausible hypothesis.

If we adopt an identity theory with regard to the relationship of physical to mental descriptions, then one further possibility is suggested by the heterostatic model. It may be noted that neuronal depolarization, hypothesized to be associated with the experience of pleasure, is an entropic process, and neuronal hyperpolarization, hypothesized to be associated with the experience of pain, is an anti-entropic process? Eddington (1958) has observed:

> The law that entropy always increases . . . holds, I think, the supreme position among the laws of Nature . . . if your theory is found to be against (it) I can give you no hope . . . From the property that entropy must always increase, practical methods of measuring it have been found. The chain of deductions from this simple law have been almost illimitable. . . . (pp. 74–75)

The possibility needs to be considered, then, that in the most general terms, entropic processes *are* pleasure and anti-entropic processes *are* pain.

If the solution of the mind-body problem requires a field phenomenon and if this field is, indeed, an electromagnetic field or a field derived from the wave properties of matter, let us now try to anticipate some of this field's properties. For example, a d-field must be followed by repolarization during the recovery process of the neuron. An h-field must be followed by partial depolarization during recovery from inhibition. Now, Eq. (18), which defines the delta value, implies that simultaneous d-fields and h-fields tend to cancel one another. If so, do the recovery processes cancel the initial depolarization or hyperpolarization of a neuron? For example, is the production of a d-field (pleasure) followed by an equal amount of pain corresponding to the repolarization? This kind of cancellation seems unlikely because, from introspection, we know that we can experience pleasure or pain continuously over extended periods of time. Introspection, therefore, suggests that the delta value does not always hover near zero. If such an observation is valid, how do we account for the wide deviations of the delta value from zero? A possible explanation is that the intensity of the pleasure or pain is proportional to the rate of change of $\Phi$. If this is true, it would eliminate the symmetry between the depolarization or hyper-polarization and the respective recovery processes, since the recovery occurs at a lower rate than the initial polarization. With the elimination of the symmetry, the cancellation of the fields would not be expected to occur.

Another property of psychic fields that we might anticipate is that the field intensity should diminish as a function of the distance from the source. This is, of course, the case with electromagnetic fields. Such would seem to be a necessary property of $\Phi$ if we are to explain the fact that the mind apparently does not reflect the state of all nearby brain structures, but only that of the MTRF.

For conscious systems other than ourselves, the information contained within the internal model that is consciousness may or may not be encoded in terms of $\Phi$, the physical variables that are identical with the psychic variables we introspectively know. Should the system's information be encoded in terms of some other set of physical phenomena, the system could *behave* as we do, but not necessarily *feel* as we do. This is a way of observing that systems may be isomorphic with respect to their behavior and still differ with respect to their psychic existence. In fact, we might ask whether there are, within the universe, relationships of a $\Phi - \Psi$ nature besides the one we are immediately concerned with here. For example, if electro-magnetic fields are the physical substrate of mental existence as we know it, might another kind of mental existence be known by a system in which other physical phenomena provided the substrate? Or if it should turn out that mental phenomena correspond to the wave aspects of matter or energy, then panpsychism would appear to become a tenable philosophy and we might have to consider the possibility of differing $\Phi - \Psi$ relationships for all material systems.

## 3.3 GLOBAL ORGANIZATION OF THE BRAIN

### 3.3.1 The Reticular Formation

The global organization of the brain can be analyzed in terms of three major subsystems: the midbrain and thalamic reticular formation (MTRF), the limbic system and hypothalamus (LSH), and the neocortex (see Figure 2). The heterostatic model suggests that each of these subsystems will seek depolarization. However, only the MTRF possesses the strategic anatomical

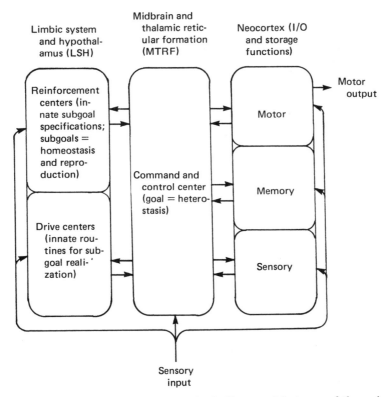

**FIGURE 2.** Global organization of the brain illustrated in terms of the major subsystems. (Direct connections between the LSH and the neocortex are not shown.)

position and connections necessary for the primary decision making role relative to the animal's total behavior. Other neural tissue may lobby, but the MTRF alone ultimately makes the decisions, and the nature of the heterostatic mechanism is such that the MTRF can decide only in favor of itself.

Having suggested that the MTRF seeks to obtain depolarization and to avoid hyperpolarization, what then are the MTRF's sources of excitation and inhibition? It is hypothesized that the sensory input channels are a principal source of excitation and that inputs mediating pain are inhibitory with respect to the MTRF. Viewing both the MTRF and the individual neuron as heterostatic systems, it is thus proposed that sensory inputs are to the MTRF what excitation is to the neuron. Similarly, pain inputs are to the MTRF what inhibition is to the neuron.

If the MTRF is a heterostat and sensory inputs, in general, are excitatory, it would be expected that animals would seek novel stimuli, since such behavior would yield positive reinforcement. (Novel stimuli are required in order to circumvent the habituation mechanism.) Of course, animals do exhibit such a drive and we term it curiosity. In the context of the heterostatic theory, therefore, curiosity is seen to be simply one route to sources of excitation for MTRF neurons. On the other hand, neuronal assemblies in the MTRF that produce behavior leading to painful stimuli will eventually become inactive because associated inhibitory transmittances will increase with each experience of pain and thus painful stimuli will be avoided.

### 3.3.2  The Limbic System and Hypothalamus

The sensory tracts and pain fibers are not the only sources of excitation and inhibition for the MTRF. Another important source is the LSH, whose principal functions appear to be that of an interface, transducer, and automatic controller located between the MTRF and the internal and external environments of the organism. The particular variables to be transduced and controlled are well known; they include temperature, heart rate and oxygen level as examples. The evolutionary process has taught the LSH to pay close attention to the essential variables of homeostasis. Specifically, it is hypothesized that the LSH, using genetically specified mechanisms, delivers generalized excitation to the MTRF (and other structures) when essential variables are moving toward homeostasis, generalized inhibition when essential variables are moving away from homeostasis, and no signal when homeostasis is obtained. This hypothesis suggests that it is the achievement of, or deviation from, homeostasis and not the maintenance of the condition that is innately reinforcing. It must be remembered that the condition of homeostasis refers to a *range* of values for the essential variables. Survival is possible so long as the variables all fall within prescribed limits. Thus, when one speaks of "moving toward homeostasis" or the "achievement of homeostasis," this usually refers to movement toward an optimal point within the prescribed limits. It can be seen that, if the MTRF is excited or inhibited by the LSH, depending on the direction of change of an animal's condition relative to homeostasis, then the MTRF will, as a consequence, seek to maintain homeostasis in its pursuit of heterostasis. Homeostasis is thus seen to be a necessary but not sufficient condition for the achievement of heterostasis.

The control function just outlined for the LSH is possibly also the mechanism responsible for producing emotions as well as such mental states as hunger and thirst. It was suggested earlier that the delivery by the LSH of generalized excitation or inhibition to the MTRF causes this conscious center to report pleasurable or painful emotional states, respectively. The specific state of the MTRF resulting from a particular configuration of excitation and inhibition impinging on it determines what emotional experience is reported. The intensity of the stimulation delivered to the MTRF determines the intensity of the emotion and also determines the magnitude of the resulting transmittance changes. Larger transmittance changes account for faster learning and more vivid memories in "emotionally charged" situations.

A more specific control function of the LSH, also accomplished with innate mechanisms, involves the generation by the LSH of specific commands appropriate to the maintenance of homeostasis. These commands result in visceral, vascular, glandular, and motor responses by the organism. It is hypothesized that what we term motivation or drive is the result of this type of LSH action. The generalized motor arousal indicating a motivated state is hypothesized to be produced by a specific facilitatory command originating within the LSH and which is sent either directly or via the MTRF to the motor cortex and, perhaps, other cortical areas. This facilitatory signal appears when there is movement away from homeostasis. The facilitation will be focused on the particular motor activities required to correct the type of deviation from homeostasis that is occurring.

The two basic LSH functions just outlined, namely, a generalized state feedback and specific reaction commands, are mediated by what may be termed *reinforcement centers* and *drive centers*, respectively. The existence of both types of centers can be demonstrated by stimulation at appropriate points within the LSH. The reinforcement centers are sometimes referred to as pleasure and pain centers. Pain centers were first observed by Delgado, Roberts, and Miller (1954). Pleasure centers were first observed by Olds and Milner (1954) in a series of self-stimulation experiments that strongly suggest the pursuit of a maximal condition as the animal's goal. Drive centers, when stimulated, produce behavior related specifically to anger, fear, or the satisfaction of hunger, thirst, or sexual needs.

It should be noted that, inasmuch as programming related to sexual needs is included in the list above, the LSH appears concerned not only with the preservation of the organism, but also with the preservation of the species. The essential variables of reproduction are assumed to be transduced and controlled in much the same manner as those associated with homeostasis.

In recent years, much knowledge has been accumulated concerning the reinforcement centers. Stein (1964a) has noted that "Largely as a result of the efforts of Olds (1962), it now seems highly probable (although direct evidence is lacking) that the hypothalamic medial forebrain bundle and its connections play a central role in the mediation of reward and that the periventricular system of the diencephalon and midbrain has a critical part in the mediation of punishment." Seven years later, Stein and Wise (1971) summarized research relating to this question:

Physiological (Olds and Milner, 1954; Olds, 1962; Miller, 1957), histochemical (Fuxe, 1965; Hillarp, Fuxe, and

Dahlstrom, 1966), and psychopharmacological (Stein and Seifter, 1961; Poschel and Ninteman, 1963; Stein, 1964b; Wise & Stein, 1969; 1970) work has led to the suggestion (Stein, 1967, 1968) that rewarded or goal-directed behavior is controlled by a specific system of norepinephrine-containing neurons in the brain. The cells of origin of this system are localized in the lower brain stem, and the axons ascend via the medial forebrain bundle to form noradrenergic synapses in the hypothalamus, limbic system, and frontal cortex. Electrical stimulation of the medial forebrain bundle serves as a powerful reward and also elicits species-typical consummatory responses, such as feeding and copulation, which produce pleasure and permit the satisfaction of basic needs (Olds and Milner, 1954; Olds, 1962; Miller, 1957). Electrolytic lesions of the medial forebrain bundle, or pharmacological blockade of its noradrenergic function, cause severe deficits in goal-directed behavior and the loss of consummatory reactions (Teitelbaum and Epstein, 1962; Hoebel, 1971). There is some evidence that these findings in animals may be extrapolated to man (Heath and Mickle, 1960; Sem-Jacobsen and Torkildsen, 1960). (p. 1032)

The portion of the lower brain stem in which the positive reinforcement neurons originate is that which Nauta (1960) has termed the limbic midbrain area (Stein, 1967). We shall enlarge our definition of the LSH so as to include this structure.

More recently, in a review of the brain reward system, Routtenberg (1978) has noted that

Since the time when the medial forebrain bundle alone was designated as the pleasure center, the boundaries of the brain reward system have been extended deep into the brain stem and far forward into the cortex of the frontal lobe of the cerebrum. All the reward systems do, however, have pathways through the medial forebrain bundle, suggesting that this region of the hypothalamus may be described as the relay station through which the brain-reward pathways course. (p. 164)

The inhibitory nature (Fuxe, 1965) of the noradrenergic positive reinforcement center outputs appears to contradict the heterostatic model proposed here where excitation is postulated to be positively reinforcing. However, Olds (1975) suggests that these noradrenergic neurons do not necessarily constitute the reward mechanism, itself, but rather may be a control mechanism that operates in conjunction with the reward mechanism. Elsewhere, Olds (1976) has suggested that "noradrenaline is in some way involved in the reward process in the normal animal, but is not the key factor in most brain-stimulation reward processes. For example, noradrenaline might be involved in the inhibitory control of negative emotional mechanisms which would themselves be incompatible with reward behavior (p. 414)." Thus, the excitatory or inhibitory nature of generalized reward mechanisms remains to be established.

An important question to consider is whether the subcortical brain can, in essence, be viewed as consisting of two functionally distinct, but highly interactive networks. The *reinforcement network*, which sets the emotional tone, might consist of the LSH reinforcement centers and the MTRF diffuse arousal system. The *drive network*, which computes the motor outputs, might consist of the LSH drive centers and the MTRF specific projection system.

The behavior of the LSH becomes more complex with time as a result of learning. The LSH, like the MTRF and other neural tissue, is assumed to undergo heterostatic adaptation. Both the reinforcement and the drive centers can, therefore, be conditioned to respond to previously neutral stimuli. A similar suggestion has been made by Stein (1964a) regarding the reinforcement centers. Stein notes that the capacity to undergo conditioning to previously neutral stimuli would provide for "activation of reinforcement systems of the brain before the occurrence of the reinforcing stimulus and is, therefore, a mechanism for anticipation or expectation (p. 117)." Stein also suggests that (1) a reciprocally inhibitory relationship exists between the reward and punishment centers, and (2) the two types of centers are continuously and jointly active in determining operant behavior. This picture of conditionable, reciprocally inhibitory, and continuously and jointly active reinforcement centers appears to be consistent with the present heterostatic theory.

With this set of assumptions, it becomes possible to understand how a nervous system could acquire conditioned defensive reflexes, as well as the appetitive reflexes already discussed. As part of the assumptions, it must be remembered that the MTRF and other structures are hypothesized to receive either excitation or inhibition from the LSH, depending on whether the animal is moving toward or away from homeostasis, and that the MTRF receives excitation from the sensory tracts and inhibition from the pain fibers. Also, the operational characteristics of the excitatory and inhibitory reinforcement centers must be kept in mind, along with the neuronal process of heterostatic adaptation. When all of these factors are considered, the acquisition of defensive conditioned reflexes can be understood in terms of an analysis like that detailed for the appetitive reflexes in Section 3.1.

### 3.3.3 The Neocortex

It is hypothesized that the relationship of the neocortex to the MTRF is as follows. When the MTRF is aroused by a stimulus, it delivers signals to the cortex, thereby facilitating cortical neurons that are also receiving the stimulus directly via the sensory tracts. The intersection of direct sensory and MTRF signals within the cortex causes some cortical neurons to fire and deliver signals back to the MTRF. In this way the MTRF, in effect, interrogates the cortex and receives a response. The response is what we subjectively interpret as sensory input or memory, depending on factors to be discussed shortly.

Another function of the MTRF signals that reach the cortex is to serve as positive reinforcement. The continual intersection of sensory and MTRF signals on cortical neurons provides the required conditions for heterostatic adaptation. In other words, *when the MTRF interrogates the cortex, it simultaneously reinforces it.* This explains the fact that what we attend to is what we remember, since it is also what is reinforced. That which is not attended to is not reinforced and, therefore, is not remembered. While cortical neurons might initially deliver a report to the MTRF only when they are driven both by sensory tract and MTRF signals, eventually, after sufficient transmittance changes occur with reinforcement, either set of signals alone may be capable of eliciting the report. For example, if one is unexpectedly confronted with a familiar face in a crowd, the cortex is capable of reporting this fact to the MTRF even though the MTRF was not specifically interrogating the cortical neurons relevant to that identification. (Some generalized facilitation of the visual cortex may have to be taking place for this pattern recognition function to occur, however.) Alternatively, a familiar face may be recalled with the delivery of appropriate signals from the MTRF to the cortex even though the person is not present and, therefore, the appropriate sensory tract signals are not available to drive the cortex. In this way, the cortical function of memory can be activated either by direct sensory stimulation of the cortex or by means of interrogation by the MTRF.

*Attention* is hypothesized to be the process whereby the MTRF selectively facilitates cortical neurons and thereby obtains specific reports from the cortex. The selective facilitation can activate sensory or memory systems. These reports, when they reach the MTRF, are interpreted as sensory inputs or memories, a distinction that is not always correctly made. For example, in the case of dreams and hallucinations, some of the information derived from memories is apparently interpreted as sensory inputs. Furthermore, Penfield (1969) has observed that when externally applied cortical stimulation activates a memory trace of a person undergoing neurosurgery, the person reports a subjective state like that associated with the original experience. The events seem to be happening again. The subjective state is not that of recall. This effect may occur because Penfield's electrode is supplying energy that would normally be supplied by impulses that reach the cortex directly via the sensory tracts. Thus, the MTRF, having received a report generated by an external energy source, may interpret the signals it is receiving as sensory input, instead of as memory. For the person undergoing the surgery, activation of the memory trace results in his experiencing two simultaneous "streams of consciousness," one associated with the sensory inputs provided by the environment of the operating room and another resulting from the external activation of the memory trace.

The act of *recall* is hypothesized to occur as follows. First, the MTRF returns to a state that is a close approximation to the state it was in when the information to be recalled was originally processed. Signals sent to the cortex from the MTRF are then similar to what they were on the previous occasion and the cortex sends back something resembling the original report. (Cortical transmittance increases make it unnecessary for the direct sensory inputs to be present this time; the signals from the MTRF are now sufficient by themselves to drive the relevant neurons.) In this way, the MTRF can become aware of, once again, what it was aware of before. We must ask, how do we retrieve the appropriate MTRF state, in the first place, in order to then elicit the desired report from the cortex? In fact, when trying to recall someone's name, for example, information about the person is already represented within the MTRF and the present MTRF state will either be the appropriate one to elicit the needed report from the cortex or the actual elicited cortical reports will drive the MTRF into the appropriate state. Should this sequence of events not occur, we will fail to recall the information. Such failures are to be expected occasionally because of the heuristic nature of the recall mechanism.

The analysis of recall just offered suggests that the retrieval of a memory only occurs in situations where the MTRF has already been driven into an appropriate state by the various signals that impinge upon it. The MTRF does not perform a search function. The inputs to the MTRF, in effect, supply the "address" for the next memory that will be called up. That is, the context within which a memory is laid down becomes the address. If a sufficient approximation to that context occurs again, as a result of the recall of another memory or due to sensory inputs, then the MTRF will automatically call up the memory laid down when the context originally occurred. Thus, memory may be viewed as a mapping of MTRF states onto the cortical "file." The brain may be said to employ a search routine as a part of its memory mechanism only to the extent that a recalled memory, in driving the MTRF into a new state, can lead to the recall of another and sometimes more relevant memory. Thus, it is hypothesized that nervous systems employ content addressable memory, a possibility that has been considered by Spinelli (1970).

A simple example may be helpful. Placing one's hand on a very hot stove may establish a memory of the event. The next time one approaches the stove, visual inputs (and other sensory cues) will drive the MTRF into a state similar to the state it was in when the hand was burned. The cortically stored memory of the previous injury will, therefore, be activated by MTRF signals (which will be similar to those sent to the cortex during the original experience) or by the direct sensory signals to the cortex, or both, and a cortical report will, therefore, reach the MTRF in time to inhibit the hand that might otherwise reach out again. The inhibitory nature of the cortical report (memory) is a consequence of the fact that pain ensued when the report was delivered to the MTRF originally, and thus reinforced inhibitory transmittances will dominate when the signals reach the MTRF again. In those cases where the inhibitory transmittances do not yet dominate, the painful act will be repeated a sufficient number of times to bring the inhibitory condition about.

In the past, the distinction between that stored information which constituted memory and that which constituted learning has been unclear or has not been made at all. The following definitions represent an attempt to distinguish the two. *Memory* is information that is acquired with cortical reinforcement supplied by the MTRF attention mechanism. *Learning* is information that is acquired with reinforcement supplied by sensory, pain fiber, or LSH activity. Memories serve the purpose, when transmitted to the MTRF, of modifying this structure's state. Memories must be stored on the input side of the MTRF, but learning can be stored on both the input and output sides. When stored on the output side, learning serves the purpose of elaborating and executing MTRF motor commands.

The dynamic processes involved in memory and learning are hypothesized to be essentially the same. Only the terminology differs. When MTRF-generated facilitation impinges upon sensory or memory cortex, we term it attention. When the facilitatory signals are directed toward motor cortex, we term it a voluntary act. In the case of memory, the MTRF signals sent to the cortex may be considered to represent a question; in the case of learning, they represent a command. If a question or command is inappropriate to present circumstances, it may result in pain, i.e., inhibition of the MTRF. This will reduce the facilitatory signals delivered to the cortex, as well as cause an increase in inhibitory transmittances associated with the generation of the question or command. Furthermore, recurrent inhibition will cause recently active cortical neurons to undergo increases in their inhibitory transmittances, insuring that the recent response will be less likely to occur in the future. On the other hand, when an appropriate response occurs, MTRF facilitation will remain, and, perhaps, even be enhanced, and recently active excitatory transmittances will increase, thereby positively reinforcing the response.

In the case of learned motor skills, when cortical excitatory transmittances become large enough, the direct signals received at the cortex from the sensory tract will, by themselves, be sufficient, or nearly so, to generate the appropriate responses. At this stage in the learning, it is necessary for the MTRF to provide only a generalized kind of facilitation to the cortex in order to initiate or maintain the appropriate activity. No longer having to issue the highly specific commands that were required during initial learning, much of the MTRF thereby becomes available to process other information, and the learned motor activity moves to a preconscious level. What has happened is that the highly specific facilitation supplied by the MTRF has been replaced, after learning, with highly specific facilitation (made so by selective transmittance increases) from the direct sensory fibers to the cortex. This explains why our awareness of activities decreases with practice of them, it becoming necessary eventually for the MTRF to issue only the generalized command (a form of facilitation) following which the learned response is executed.

In this discussion of the neocortex, it ought to be noted that this structure contains innate as well as acquired information-processing capabilities. In the case of the cat's visual cortex, for example, Hubel and Wiesel (1965) have shown that at least up to the level of the striate cortex, the functional organization is genetically specified. Thus, when a newborn kitten first interrogates the visual cortex, it is receiving more than "raw" sensory inputs. Presumably, innate preprocessors of this kind also occur in other cortical areas.

One relationship that we have not yet considered is that of the LSH to the neocortex. Does the LSH directly reinforce the neocortex in the same way that it has been hypothesized to directly reinforce the MTRF? Other questions can also be posed. Do some of the various specialized commands issued by the LSH for the maintenance of homeostasis go directly to the cerebral cortex or does the motor arousal associated with a motivated state, for example, result from signals sent indirectly via the MTRF? Does the neocortex supply sensory and memory inputs directly to the LSH? At this point, specific conjectures will not be offered regarding these issues. Such conjectures would take us too far afield and are not essential to the further development of other aspects of the present theory.

### 3.3.4  Vector Specification of the Brain State

If we wish to characterize the state of a nervous system in a concise manner, given that the neural connectivity pattern has already been specified, we might do so with the specification of two vectors. The MTRF-state vector has already been defined. This vector specifies the dynamic state of the command and control center and thereby displays our state of conscious awareness. We might define a second vector and term it the *weight* or *transmittance vector*. This vector will have one component for each synapse in the nervous system, each component specifying the corresponding synaptic transmittance. The vector is, therefore, a way of representing the state of memory and learning of the organism. If the human nervous system contains $10^{12}$ neurons and the average neuron receives, perhaps $10^4$ synapses, then the transmittance vector for a person will be a $10^{16}$-tuple. In time, with the accumulation of memories and the occurrence of learning, this transmittance vector comes to represent an increasingly accurate model of the person, the person's environment and his or her relationship to that environment. Utilizing the information, it eventually becomes possible for the MTRF to make accurate predictions, to discover new relationships among those relationships already known, and to seek answers to questions regarding its own fundamental nature.

## 3.4  SOME FURTHER OBSERVATIONS

### 3.4.1  Memory and Learning

One of the characteristics of brain function that has seemed most remarkable has been the distributed nature of memory and learning within the cortex. This feature is understandable in light of the global organization proposed above. The MTRF is continuously broadcasting signals to large portions of the cortex. In order to interrogate a memory or initiate a learned response, the MTRF must at least approximately reproduce the signal configuration employed when the memory or learned response was initially established. No aspect of the proposed mechanism makes it necessary for the MTRF to utilize contiguous cortical neurons for these functions. When a memory is retrieved or a motor act is executed, it would appear to be as easy to signal a widely distributed collection of neurons as it would a localized collection. In fact, with the kind of global organization proposed, a localized memory might be difficult to obtain. Thus, the proposed storage and recall mechanism makes plausible the distributed nature of memory and learning.

That the storage may be highly redundant is also plausible. In effect, the function of the cortex, upon receiving a signal configuration from the MTRF, is to deliver a set of signals that will produce an appropriate motor response or drive the MTRF into a new state that represents recalled or sensory information. When a memory is established or learning has occurred, there is no reason to believe that only the required minimum number of cortical neurons will have their synaptic transmittances modified. In fact, it may be that large redundancies are difficult to avoid. Thus, the continued successful function of the brain is plausible in spite of the localized destruction of tissue in the case of injury or disease.

It is also possible to understand the recovery of function observed after extensive damage to the nervous system, especially in a young animal. Due to the localized neural process of heterostatic adaptation, when the structure of the nervous system is altered due to damage, the individual neurons that survive will readjust, seeking once more to maximize the amount of polarization they can obtain from the new signal configurations they will be receiving. This readjustment and the observed recovery of function are hypothesized to be one and the same process.

Concerning the difference between short-term memory (STM) and long-term memory (LTM), it seems likely that STM consists of active feedback loops between the MTRF and other structures, principally the cortex. STM is, therefore, reflected in the MTRF state vector. LTM, on the other hand, consists of the modified transmittance values of cortical and other neurons and, thus, is reflected in the transmittance vector.

A feedback relationship, similar to that proposed between the neocortex and the MTRF, may also be expected to exist between the MTRF and other brain structures; memory and learning are not the exclusive domain of the neocortex, although this structure is clearly highly advanced in regard to these functions. The extent of these feedback loops between the MTRF and other structures may correlate with their observed epileptogenicity, which is to say, their tendency to give rise to convulsions. It was noted in Chapter 2 that Goddard, using a novel stimulation technique, found that an epileptic focus could be established in the amygdala within 15 days, but none was established in the reticular formation after 200 days of stimulation. Goddard's stimulation of various sites within the brain may have resulted in the activation of MTRF-mediated feedback loops that, in turn, supplied a further polarizing bias to the stimulated area. If this kind of reinforcing feedback is occurring during the development of an epileptic focus, epileptogenicity will tend to be proportional to the extensiveness of the feedback loops between the stimulated area and the MTRF.

The extensive feedback loops that exist between the two cortical hemispheres may contribute to the epileptogenicity of the cerebral cortex. That such loops are involved in some cases of epilepsy is suggested by the fact that surgical separation of the two hemispheres has produced marked improvement in severely epileptic patients (Sperry 1966; Gazzaniga, 1970).

Are painful memories most easily forgotten? This is reasonable if, because of conditioning, the LSH reacts to the memory as it did to the original experience. The LSH may then be expected to inhibit the MTRF activity involved in the recall and, thus, this MTRF state is less likely to occur again. Forgetting, in this case, refers to a loss of the ability to retrieve the cortically stored memory. With regard to the general question of whether forgetting is due to interference or decay of memory traces, the neuronal model and global brain organization proposed here renders interference highly plausible, but offers no basis for the occurrence of memory trace decay. This appears to be consistent with the psychological evidence on the question.

### 3.4.2 Pleasure and Pain

Hilgard (1969), in a paper entitled "Pain as a Puzzle for Psychology and Physiology," raised four fundamental questions regarding the nature of pain. We will try to answer them now on the basis of the proposed theory.

*"Is pain a sensory modality?"* It is not, no more than pleasure is. Both the experience of pleasure and that of pain can, at times, be highly correlated with activity within sensory tracts or "pain fibers," when these are delivering excitation or inhibition to the MTRF. At other times, however, the source of the excitation or inhibition is the LSH and then the subjective experience is that of diffuse and internally generated sensations that we describe as emotions. The intensity of pleasure or pain has already been suggested to be approximately proportional to the delta value [see Eq. (18)]. The specific subjective experience, whether of vision, audition, touch, joy, grief, anger, fear, etc., depends on the specific configuration of depolarizing and hyperpolarizing events occurring within the MTRF. It is expected that we place subjective experiences in the same or different categories, depending on the extent of similarity between the respective MTRF state vectors. In terms of the reinforcement and drive networks of the LSH, the former sets the emotional tone while the latter accomplishes specific computations of motor commands and, also, the retrieval of memories to be utilized in computing future motor commands.

Hilgard notes that "any stimulus can qualify to produce pain if it is intense enough." This fact suggests that, with increasing intensity, all stimuli eventually become inhibitory with respect to the MTRF.

The relief from intense pain that is obtained with frontal lobe operations suggests that feedback loops between the MTRF and the frontal lobes have the effect of sustaining or even amplifying inhibition occurring within the MTRF. The relief from anxiety (assumed here to be an inhibition-dominant MTRF state) that is obtained after prefrontal lobotomy further suggests an important relationship between the frontal lobes and MTRF inhibition.

*"Are there any satisfactory physiological indicators of pain?"* None have been found, as Hilgard notes, and none are likely to be discovered. Within the MTRF, the complex interplay between excitation and inhibition that corresponds to the subjective experiences of pleasure and pain should not be expected to correlate reliably with any physiological indicator. The inhibition that is experienced as pain by the MTRF might well result from a complex interplay of excitatory and inhibitory neural activity nearer to the sensory surface. Melzack and Wall's (1965) gate-control theory of pain, much discussed in recent years, is an attempt to deal with such complexities. A recent critical review of this theory is provided by Nathan (1976).

*"Where is the pain that is felt?"* It is within the MTRF, along with everything else of which we are said to possess conscious awareness. The projection to a location on the body is accomplished with information that is probably obtained from the regular sensory channels.

Is is interesting to note that, in the case of phantom-limb pain, the projected location doesn't even exist. Prior to the loss of the limb the projection of sensations to that location on the body may have been learned. Alternatively, such projections may be genetically specified. In either case, the phenomenon of phantom-limb pain may arise because the amounts of excitation and inhibition being delivered to the MTRF from a given part of the body are normally in a state of balance—a state that may be disturbed when the peripheral nervous system is altered.

*"How account for the great individual differences in felt*

*pain?"* This is understandable when one realizes that pain is not something as narrow in scope as a sensory modality. Pleasure and pain are the two fundamental currencies with which all of the nervous system's transactions are carried out. The great individual differences in felt pain reflect the genetic and experiential differences among people. It is reasonable that many aspects of nervous system function should influence the subjective experience of pain, because we are really talking about a phenomenon as pervasive as inhibition. The variability among people in their reaction to pain is paralleled by the variability of results obtained by the neurosurgeon when he operates to relieve pain. This type of surgery does not always produce clear-cut, reliable results. As with the sources of inhibition, the sources of pain are multiple and complex.

Having reviewed the questions raised by Hilgard, several other observations may be made before leaving the subject of pleasure and pain. Fear may be considered to be the memory of inflicted pain. The memory can be of genetic origin (in which case we are using the term "memory" in a much wider sense than usual) or it may be acquired. An animal will "freeze" in a situation that produces extreme fear. This may be a consequence of massive inhibition occurring within the MTRF. Also consistent with the proposed theory, pleasurable circumstances reveal an excited MTRF—people feel like "dancing in the street."

On the battlefield (and ,the playing field), people can be observed with severe injuries and, yet, they may experience no pain. Apparently, the inhibition being delivered to the MTRF, as great as it is, is overwhelmed by the massive excitation simultaneously delivered by the LSH in the heat of the battle. This is a circumstance where the two terms in Eq. (18), $Q(D)$ and $Q(H)$, are both very large. A positive delta value results because the fight mechanism of the LSH is assumed to supply large amounts of excitation. (This assumption that the innate LSH fight mechanism is a source of excitation and, therefore, of pleasure for the MTRF may also, in part, explain man's tendency to undertake wars.) If the flight mechanism takes over and delivers inhibition to the MTRF, causing $Q(H)$ to increase, or the contest ends causing $Q(D)$ to decrease, then the delta value becomes negative and pain is experienced. Roughly speaking, it can be seen that Eq. (18) is to the whole animal what inequality (7) is to the neuron.

An important observation concerning pain is that we do not habituate to it. This is consistent with the fact that no mechanism has been observed that relates to the inhibitory neurons in the way that the feed-forward and recurrent inhibition hypothesized to underly habituation relate to excitatory neurons. Perhaps the system evolved this way because the ability to habituate to pleasurable stimuli and the inability to habituate to painful simuli both have survival value.

One final comment of a general nature may be in order regarding pleasure and pain. If the heterostatic theory is correct, behavioral psychologists can take a broader view of positive and negative reinforcement because the theory extends the behavioral psychologist's paradigm to include the single neuron as well as the whole organism. Many experimenters who have sought to condition single neurons have assumed as much for years. However, they have done so without examining the theoretical implications of such an implicit heterostatic view of neuronal function.

The heterostatic theory leads to the view that essentially all stimuli are reinforcing, at least for advanced organisms. Stimuli that produce clear-cut reinforcing effects probably do so because they are transformed by the LSH into large amounts of either excitation or inhibition that "washes over" controlling neurons. All other stimuli produce more complex patterns of excitation and inhibition that do not yield such clear reinforcing effects at the level of the whole organism. But these stimuli are probably reinforcers, nonetheless. In these more complex cases, we must consider the possibility that neurons are being reinforced more or less locally and individually, some positively and some negatively. It has probably been a mistake to assume that most stimuli play only a "neutral," information bearing, nonreinforcing role. In the heterostatic theory, all stimuli are seen to have dual roles, serving both as bearers of information in a more neutral, open-loop sense and as reinforcers. This may help to explain the complications that confront the behavioral psychologists when they apply their theory in practical social situations.

### 3.4.3 Sleep and Dreaming

Sleep and dreaming are complex phenomena that are not yet well understood. Their functions, the mechanisms involved and the nature of possible associated regulatory centers remain unclear. In this difficult situation, some conjectures based on the MTRF hypothesis and the postulated heterostatic adaptive mechanism may be helpful.

Assuming the human MTRF is a conscious command and control center consisting of heterostatic neurons, we may consider how this center might become organized as it acquires experience. Initially, which is to say, around the time of birth, control might be shared more or less equally among all of the neurons within the MTRF. However, those neurons whose firing results in punishment will become increasingly inhibited due to the heterostatic adaptive mechanism. Thus, as the MTRF accumulates experience, a generally inhibited subset of neurons will develop. The remaining neurons will constitute a generally active subset that will control behavior. The boundary between the two subsets will necessarily vary with time, depending on immediate inputs and the present pattern of activity within the MTRF.

Sleep researchers have not yet established that sleep has a restorative function. However, having conjectured that our MTRF becomes divided into generally active and generally inhibited neural subsets, let us consider what the system dynamics of the MTRF might be if the active neurons are subject to "fatigue." To consider a hypothetical example, suppose the firing of a neuron over a period of time temporarily depletes its supply of transmitter substance. If this or some other process leading to fatigue occurs, then the active neural subset will need to shut down periodically so that a restorative process can take place. Such a cessation of activity or sleep may occur under the partial control of an evolved "sleep center" that coordinates the sleep-waking cycle. We can see that during sleep the possibility arises of the usually inhibited neural subset becoming active. Such activity seems likely for two reasons. First, a primary source of the subset's inhibition is expected to be the usually active neural subset, now "asleep." Secondly, neurons in the usually inhibited subset will not be fatigued because they will not have been firing much or at all during the waking period. The stage is thus set for the emergence of a *dreaming subset* of MTRF neurons that is active when the animal is asleep, along with a *waking subset* of MTRF neurons that is active and in control when the animal is awake. Some of the characteristic activity patterns that would be expected of an MTRF organized in this way may now be considered.

In general, the brain does not become inactive during sleep. However, what is sometimes termed the "arousal system" does cease its activity (Moruzzi and Magoun, 1949). This has prompted some researchers to conclude that the arousal system *causes* wakefulness. It seems more likely that the activity of the arousal system *is* wakefulness. If the arousal system is part of the conscious command and control center of the brain, as suggested earlier, we can understand why this structure would need rest when much of the remainder of the brain might not.

Probably no portion of the brain bears so constant a load during waking hours as the MTRF. While other brain structures might well be able to carry out their recovery processes during waking hours, such is less likely to be the case for the waking MTRF. It becomes understandable, for example, that an extreme lack of sleep should lead to hallucinations and mild delusions, this being consistent with the idea of a fatigued waking MTRF whose neurons have become increasingly unresponsive for the lack of a recovery period.

If sleep is recovery from MTRF fatigue, which is a consequence of extended neuronal firing, then the amount of sleep required will depend on the information processing load put on the MTRF. Such a correlation seems to be borne out by the evidence. The amount of sleep needed appears to increase with the amount of learning occurring during the day and also as the amount of stress or worry increases (Hartmann, 1973). That some degree of apparent recovery can be accomplished simply by changing activities is reasonable because different activities would likely involve different (though possibly over-lapping) cell assemblies.

The information processing load placed on the MTRF during learning can be appreciated through introspection. When learning to drive a car, for example, one observes that consciousness is almost fully occupied with the business of driving. However, as learning occurs (assumed here to be, in effect, the laying down of cortical "subroutines)," the load on conscious control diminishes (because cortical cell assemblies acquire the ability to compute the appropriate motor responses directly). After one has learned to drive, the MTRF need only decide to drive to a particular place and then to a large degree the cortical cell assemblies take over, leaving the conscious MTRF free to think about, or work on, other things. In this context, learning is seen to be a kind of habituation of the MTRF as the cortex takes over the learned function.

That the waking MTRF lapses into sleep out of boredom as well as fatigue seems reasonable. Because of the very nature of the waking MTRF, it is likely to be dependent on a steady stream of inputs to drive it from state to state in what has been termed the "stream of consciousness." Should the MTRF be receiving inputs largely of kinds to which it has already habituated, it may lapse into non-activity leading to sleep. In such circumstances, sleep would seem even more likely if the MTRF's relationship to an evolved sleep center is one of reciprocal inhibition. Inactivity on the part of the MTRF would then permit arousal of the sleep center.

According to the relationship we have hypothesized, when the waking MTRF is most thoroughly shut down for rest, the dreaming MTRF is most likely to be active. Because dreams are known to be associated with rapid eye movement or REM (Dement and Kleitman, 1957), it is appropriate to examine some of the attributes of REM sleep to determine if they are consistent with the attributes we would expect of the dreaming MTRF.

The MTRF might be expected to oscillate in and out of the dream state, as appears to be the case, because activity in the dreaming MTRF may well recruit more and more neurons in the waking MTRF until the waking MTRF's activity significantly inhibits the dreaming MTRF and shuts it down again. Also, if REM sleep is associated with an inactive waking MTRF that is undergoing a recovery process, then the amount of REM sleep required should increase as the information processing load on the waking MTRF increases. Such appears to be the case both from a phylogenetic and an ontogenetic standpoint. Hartmann (1966) notes that REM sleep does not occur at all in the lowest animals, but increases to about 25% for mammals. This seems reasonable in light of the extensive "auxiliary processors" (the LSH and neocortex) that the MTRF must interact with in mammals. The percentage of REM sleep is greatest at birth and during childhood and then declines with adulthood. This would seem to correlate with the information processing load expected to be associated with learning during childhood.

Deprivation of REM sleep by waking a subject whenever he goes into a REM period is disturbing to the subject and produces irritability (Dement, 1960). This effect is not seen when an equal number of interruptions of sleep occur during non-REM periods. This can be understood in terms of the waking MTRF and the expected effect on it of interruptions of its recovery periods. In accordance with the hypotheses stated above, it would be during REM sleep that the waking MTRF would be most quiet and thus have the best opportunity to recover from its high level of waking activity. Interruptions of REM sleep may, therefore, interfere with the waking MTRF's recovery process. This is consistent with the observation that REM percentage rebounds after suppression (Dement, 1960), indicating that the waking MTRF must necessarily have a certain percentage of "down time" for the recuperative processes to occur.

Interruptions of REM sleep would also be expected to facilitate the waking MTRF's awareness and memory of an ongoing dream if the relevant MTRF and cortical neurons, whose activity relate to the dream, continue to be active for a short time while the waking MTRF is being aroused. Thus, the waking MTRF has a brief opportunity to access the dream in a way that it could not normally. Usually, when the waking MTRF is active, the dreaming MTRF is inactive, along with, perhaps, most of the cortical cell assemblies that are especially aroused by the dreaming MTRF. Probable overlap of cortical cell assemblies accessed by the waking and dreaming MTRF's would explain the ability most of us have to partially recall dream content. Also, by interrupting REM sleep regularly and recording dream content, one might increase the overlap of cortical cell assemblies (memory) that can be accessed by both the waking and dreaming MTRF, thus producing a greater capability for dream recall.

Introspectively established characteristics of dreams are also understandable in terms of the nature of the dreaming MTRF. Because the dreaming MTRF would appear to be a product of inhibitory reinforcement, it is understandable that dream content often reflects repressed behavior and ideas. It is reasonable that such dream content might be expressed in a disorganized and sometimes bizarre fashion because the neurally represented negations in the dreaming MTRF have no opportunity to become well organized with respect to one another; they are simply isolated fragments of negatively reinforced aspects of reality. That positively reinforced aspects of reality are also reflected in dreams is probably due to participation by neural assemblies from the waking MTRF. Such participation might be expected from neurons that fired little or not at all during waking hours. The absence of fatigue in these neurons probably makes them vulnerable to recruiting by the dreaming MTRF either directly or indirectly through other brain structures. Also, other brain structures that were activated during waking hours and continued their activity into sleep could be responsible for recruiting MTRF neurons for participation during a dream, thus providing a basis for some correlation between dream content and recent waking activity.

It seems likely that, during dreaming, neural activity patterns within the MTRF will occur that make no sense at all. If such happens, they would never be reported by a waking MTRF simply because their incoherence would probably render their recall impossible.

We have considered the MTRF as a conscious command and control center that, through experience, develops into two parts, a waking and a dreaming MTRF. If this is so, it would appear that in some sense we are all "split personalities" and, in fact, this proposed view of MTRF function suggests the basis of an explanation for the seemingly bizarre phenomenon of the multiple personality.

The dreaming MTRF has been hypothesized to be a

collection of punished behaviors and ideas. Suppose, in unusual circumstances, that some additional specific set of cohering behaviors and ideas were to be consistently negatively rein- forced such as, for example, a particular set of personality attributes. It seems conceivable that in such a case, if conditions were extreme, a third subset of MTRF cell assemblies might develop with respect to one another and they could represent, for example, a "forbidden" personality. When the waking MTRF was in control, it would then be inhibiting two other neural subsets, the dreaming MTRF and what might be called the *split MTRF*. (In some cases, there might be more than one split MTRF.) The waking MTRF might have no more, and maybe even less knowledge of the split MTRF than it does of the dreaming MTRF because of the impossibility of accessing the relevant information. However, if on waking on some mornings, the split MTRF were to take control because of chance patterns of neural acitivity, it might conceivably possess some awareness of the waking MTRF because strong inhibitions from the split MTRF to the waking MTRF would not be so likely. If there were sufficient reciprocal inhibition between the waking and split MTRF's, then only one could be in control at any given time. The one that gained control at the onset of wakefulness might retain control all day. Only its shutting down for sleep would provide an opportunity for the other neural subset to gain control when wakefulness occurred again.

### 3.4.4 Nature of Man

The present theory suggests a very simple and very old answer to a basic philosophical question. What is the fundamental nature of man? Man is a hedonist (a form of heterostat). Many of the implications of a hedonistic view of human behavior are well discussed by Campbell (1973). Probably most, if not all, other forms of advanced animal life are hedonists also.

The conclusion that man is a hedonist has been rejected by many in the past for three scientific reasons. First, definitions of pleasure and pain in other than behavioral terms were lacking. Second, no underlying neurophysiological mech- anism was apparent that would support such a thesis. Third, our behavior appears to be truly altruistic at times (discounting the occasions when apparent altruism is only a ploy). The proposed neuronal model suggests answers to the first two objections.

To meet the third objection, a new hypothesis must be introduced. It is proposed that the LSH has a capacity for distinguishing between self and other, but that it is severely limited. Specifically, it is proposed that our LSH is a primitive brain that (in conjunction with the MTRF) simply regards people as "others" if the fight-fright-flight drive centers are active, but otherwise does not distinguish between other and self. This conjecture, which will be termed the *LSH hypothesis*, is supported by evidence drawn from human behavior. For example, our aversion to killing other humans decreases as the relevant sensory stimuli diminish. The strong inhibition is present only when the LSH, driven by appropriate sensory inputs, can (mistakenly) interpret the situation as self-injurious. A bomber pilot can knowingly produce immense suffering and death from the cockpit, whereas he might well be rendered psychotic if he had to accomplish the same amount of destruction of life while he was face-to-face with his victims. Remove the relevant sensory input and the inhibition against inflicting pain or death upon another human diminishes, although not usually to zero because the cortical functions of memory and learning provide approximations to the relevant sensory inputs when they are not present. In addition, most cultures have, to some degree, conditioned their members not to harm other humans.

Further evidence of the inability of the LSH to make the self-other distinction is provided by an observation that Lorenz (1970) has discussed. Humans find it increasingly difficult to kill animals as their *external* resemblance to humans increases. In order of increasing difficulty, Lorenz mentions fish, frogs ("it is the humanlike arms and legs of these creatures that render their slaughtering so odious, though from the point of view of neural and 'mental' development they are vastly inferior to the higher fish"), dogs, and monkeys.

That the LSH tends to incorporate the other into the self, except under fight-fright-flight circumstances, is also evidenced by the fact that the amount of seemingly altruistic behavior exhibited by an individual is a function of the extent to which he or she is acquainted with the other person or animal. Lorenz (1970) has noted that researchers experience increased difficulty in sacrificing a laboratory animal if the animal has been known to them for a relatively long period of time. The difficulties increase further if the animal has required considerable care.

The present context is, perhaps, an appropriate one in which to consider the psychological concepts of love and hatred. Hatred would appear to be a psychological state in which the fight-fright-flight drive centers are active and, thus, the LSH is capable of making the self-other distinction. Love, on the other hand, is hypothesized to be a psychological state in which the LSH does not make the self-other distinction. If this is true, then "Love thy neighbor as thyself" assumes the nature, in part, of a definition.

The innate decision-making processes of the LSH are supplemented in humans by much learned behavior. The question arises as to whether the greater ability of our highly educated cortex to assist the MTRF in making distinctions between self and other has increased our aggressiveness as compared to that of the other primates. It would seem that learning can either support or oppose the innate processes of the LSH. If, for example, people are taught prejudicial attitudes toward another group of people, those persons will perceive less of a resemblance between themselves and members of the other group. The increased ease in making the self-other distinction increases the likelihood that people will behave detrimentally toward those against whom they have been prejudiced. On the other hand, an educational process that reveals the similarities among all persons will support and strengthen behavior that is a consequence of the LSH's identification of self and other.

### 3.4.5 Epistemology

The neuron is a cell in pursuit of excitation. At the level of the whole person, this neuronal goal reveals itself, in part, as the pursuit of knowledge or, more generally, the pursuit of stimulation. Of crucial importance in this process is the habituation mechanism. Without it, redundant stimuli could satisfy the neuron. Novel stimuli would not be sought, knowledge would not be acquired, and the survival of the species would be unlikely.

In the context of the present theory, knowledge is a collection of causal relations encoded in the form of synaptic transmittance values. Transmittances are measures of the likelihood that excitation or inhibition will follow if the neuron responds when the associated synapses are active. Thus, at the level of the neuron, information is encoded in a simple, direct form. Impulses reach the neuron as weighted advice to fire or not to fire—nothing more. It is only from the viewpoint of the whole brain that strings of excitatory and inhibitory impulses take on more complex meanings.

# Chapter 4
# cybernetics

Cybernetic research into adaptive and intelligent systems has usually assumed one of two forms. The adaptive network approach, characterized by a microscopic, neurophysiological orientation, grew out of the early work of investigators such as Rashevsky (1938) and McCulloch and Pitts (1943). The alternative approach of artificial intelligence, with its macroscopic, psychological orientation, developed out of the work of investigators such as Newell, Shaw, and Simon (1957, 1958) and Samuel (1959). Some cyberneticians, such as Wiener (1948) and Ashby (1952), have influenced researchers of both orientations. In this chapter, we will examine the relationship of the present theory to both approaches and will then consider possible directions for future research.

Artificial intelligence research is generally defined so as to include adaptive network research. However, such a definition can blur fundamental distinctions. To view adaptive networks as a part of artificial intelligence can be as confusing as it would be to view neurophysiology as a part of psychology. The very real differences between adaptive network and most other artificial intelligence researchers are reflected in the basic assumptions of the two groups. Adaptive network researchers have generally believed that the fundamental mechanisms underlying intelligence reside, at least in part, at a level corresponding to that of the single neuron. Most artificial intelligence researchers, on the other hand, work at a much higher level, with the view that the nature of the component at the level of the single neuron is not of theoretical significance, for their purposes. In recognition of these fundamentally different assumptions and approaches, adaptive network and artificial intelligence research will be treated separately in this chapter.

## 4.1  ADAPTIVE NETWORKS

In the construction and simulation of adaptive networks for experimental purposes, usually one of two types of connection-istic neuronal models has been employed. In one type, which will be designated as the Type I or *association model*, it is assumed that the repetitive activation of a synapse, when this contributes to the firing of the recipient neuron, is the basis for increasing the effectiveness of the synapse. Hebb (1949) adopted this assumption in developing his theory of cell assemblies. Eccles (1964), in a review, notes that variations of this assumption have been considered by Tanzi (1893), Ramon y Cajal (1911), Konorski (1948, 1950), Tonnees (1949), Young (1951), Eccles (1953), Jung (1953), McIntyre (1953), and Thorpe (1956). Hebb's theory provided the basis for further research by Rochester et al. (1956), Milner (1957), Good (1965), Finley (1967), Sampson (1969), Marr (1969), and Cunningham (1972), among others. Uttley (1966, 1975), guided by the notion of "local efficiency," has extended Hebb's model by investigating a network in which the contribution of a neuronal input is made proportional to the Shannon information between that input and the neuronal output. More recently, Uttley (1976a, 1976b, 1976c) has extended these results for the case in which every adaptive neuron, during the training phase, receives nonadaptive co-occurring "classifying" inputs that provide an immediate indication of whether a neuronal response is desirable. In these studies, Uttley proposes that the transmittance of a variable synapse becomes proportional to the negative of the Shannon mutual information function between the neuron's inputs and output.

Association models of the neuron are based on the assumption that adaptive changes are a function of co-occurring neuronal events. A classical conditioning orientation is implicit in such models. With *reinforcement models*, on the other hand, an instrumental conditioning orientation is adopted; it is assumed that sequential rather than simultaneous events are of fundamental importance. Neuronal models are then investigated in which adaptive changes are a function of reinforcement signals received after neuronal responses. With this type of model, which will be designated as Type II, the dynamic, temporal aspects of biological information processing are seen as a cause-effect chaining of sequences rather than as the ongoing detection of simultaneous events.

Whether, in fact, sequentiality or simultaneity rules the single neuron remains for future experimental work to determine. At this point, however, Type I (association) models do not look promising. The inadequacy of association models of neuronal function has been analyzed by Sutton and Barto (1979). For example, with regard to neuronal models like that proposed by Hebb (1949), Sutton and Barto conclude:

> While the spirit of Hebb's theory still seems to be relevant, there is little support for the use of a literal interpretation of the Hebbian rule in adaptive network studies. As a model of classical conditioning, it is not up to the standard of sophistication now readily available in the learning theory literature. As a model of neural plasticity, it lacks experimental support and is based on a view of the processing capabilities of neurons and synapses which does not take into account the wealth of data now available. While networks employing the Hebbian rule have been successful in producing some interesting effects, their behavior is far from the level of sophistication required for complex tasks as evidenced by the general abandonment of their study within the field of Artificial Intelligence. Finally, models relying on the Hebbian rule require rather ad hoc additional mechanisms to insure stable and flexible behavior.

The neuronal model proposed in the present theory belongs to the Type II category. Type II neuronal models were first employed in adaptive networks developed by Minsky (1954) and Farley and Clark (1954). Variations of the Type II model have been employed in the extensive investigations of perceptrons initiated by Rosenblatt (1957, 1962) and also in studies by Selfridge (1959), Palmieri and Sanna (1960), Gamba et al. (1961), Widrow (1962), Widrow and Hoff (1960), and Widrow et al., (1963), Brain et al. (1963), Kaylor (1964), and Klopf (1971), among others. Type II neuronal models can be further categorized in accordance with whether they employ "restricted" or "generalized" reinforcement signals. The Type II models referenced above may be described as *restricted reinforcement models*. In these cases the neuron is viewed as the recipient of three or four different signal types, these signals being excitation and inhibition along with special reward and/ or punishment inputs. The assumption that the neuronal reinforcement signals are of a special restricted nature, different at least in effect from the other excitatory and inhibitory inputs, creates a wide division between the "teacher" (the source of the reinforcement signals) and the remainder of the adaptive system and environment. These restricted reinforcement models have not led to large, powerful adaptive networks, probably because of the extent of their reliance on global reinforcement mechanisms.

In contrast to restricted reinforcement models, the proposed heterostatic neuronal model exemplifies *generalized reinforcement,* where all (or at least many) input signals are potential reinforcers. In the heterostatic theory, a special teacher—the LSH, for example—may provide reinforcement, but environmental stimuli may more directly do so. Sensory inputs may be rewarding (e.g., excitation delivered to the MTRF) or punishing (e.g., inhibition delivered to the MTRF). In addition, the signals transmitted between neural structures may be reinforcing, as in the case of selective MTRF facilitation of the cortex resulting in our remembering that to which we attend.

Historically, viewing the neuron as a goal-seeking element goes back to the work of Freud (1895). Freud proposed that CNS neurons, in their "primary function" seek to minimize the amount of excitation received. Freud also suggested that a "secondary process" occurred that maintained a low, steady-state level of excitation required for basic processes such as respiration. Cybernetic research into generalized goal-seeking neuronal models originated with Griffith's proposal (1962, 1963) for a network element that minimized a "power function" of its inputs and output. Subsequently, Wilkins (1970) proposed a neuron that sought to minimize the "total information exchange during a computation. . . . consistent with the computation." Neuronal models like those proposed by Griffith and Wilkins will have to be thoroughly understood if we are to develop a general theory of adaptive networks. However, the apparent appetite of the single neuron and the whole organism for positive reinforcement is not consistent with Griffith's and Wilkins' views of living systems as minimizers.

At a time when the present book was nearly completed, the author learned of one other view of the neuron as a goal-seeker. Based on his study of infantile autism, Rimland (1964) suggested that "behavior might very well be defined in terms of an organism's efforts toward attempting to maximize . . . intra-neuronal reward." Rimland proposed that "neurons seek stimula-tion" or, alternatively, that "neurons 'want' to discharge" and he associated this neuronal pursuit with our experience of pleasure. Rimland did not propose an adaptive mechanism for such a neuron. However, it is clear that he anticipated the explanatory power of such an approach. Thus, Rimland appears to have been the first investigator to consider the possibility that neurons are hedonists.

For the reader who desires more than the very brief historical review presented here, Arbib (1975a) has surveyed adaptive net-work research and, in a review of the relationship of artificial intel-ligence to brain theory, Arbib (1975b) has discussed goal-seeking in the context of "cooperative computation." In addition, the bib-liographic notes of Nilsson (1965) and Minsky and Papert (1969) provide overviews of the literature of adaptive network studies.

We may now summarize the differences in point of view and assumptions between a generalized reinforcement model such as the heterostat and most previous work in adaptive network research. The problem of understanding adaptive networks has usually been viewed from the top down rather than from the bottom up. That is to say, the tendency has been to think in terms of the *system* goals and then ask what network structure and mechanisms would permit these goals to be realized. The viewpoint of the heterostatic theory is the opposite. A goal is assumed for the individual network elements and then behavior of the total system is analyzed in terms of this elemental goal. From a theoretical point of view, the two approaches can be equivalent, of course. However, the perspective that results is very different, depending on whether one focuses on the system goals first and the elemental behavior second or on an elemental goal first and the consequent system behavior second. For the general case of goal-seeking adaptive networks of goal-seeking adaptive components, both viewpoints will, of course, always have to be kept in mind. However, in the case of biological systems, the bottom-up viewpoint ought to be especially appropriate because it corresponds to the way in which living systems evolved.

In reviewing different approaches to adaptive networks, it is of interest to compare statistical versus deterministic adaptive mechanisms. The proposed heterostatic theory assumes that nervous systems employ a statistical adaptive process, a process in which the chance occurrence of appropriate or inappropriate behavior is rewarded or punished, respectively. It is hypothesized that such a mechanism produces a network that tends to model the organism and the environment. As the model becomes increasingly refined, the statistical aspect of the adaptive process becomes less important and behavior becomes more directed. In contrast to this type of mechanism, much adaptive network research has assumed a deterministic adaptive process. This assumption grew out of the discovery of the perceptron convergence theorem (Rosenblatt, 1960), which provides an algorithmic adaptive procedure. Such a mechanism has many advantages. However, the algorithm applies only to single-layered adaptive networks. Much subsequent research has failed to produce a truly viable deterministic adaptive mechanism for the more general case of the multilayer network. The central problem in the general case is that of establishing what any given network element *should* be doing when the system behavior is inappropriate. This has proved very difficult because most of the outputs of individual elements in a deep network bear a highly indirect relationship to the final output of the system. It should be noted that the discovery of the convergence theorem did not cause Rosenblatt to rely exclusively on a global adaptive process. He continued to believe that local adaptive processes were of fundamental importance, an assumption that was adopted in formulating the present theory.

## 4.2  ARTIFICIAL INTELLIGENCE

For two decades now, artificial intelligence (AI) researchers have sought increasingly powerful information processing systems and better models of intelligence through the development of new forms of software, sensors, and effectors for the digital computer. For an introduction to this research, the reader should consult the collections of papers edited by Feigenbaum and Feldman (1963) and Minsky (1969). In addition, a survey by Nilsson (1974) provides an excellent review of the field and, more recently, Boden (1979) has surveyed the field from a more humanistic perspective.

In recent years, AI research has frequently been assessed in terms of such questions as whether the research has accomplished much, what in principle can be accomplished, who should accomplish it, and whether AI is dangerous (see, for example, Dreyfus, 1965, 1972; Lighthill, 1973; Roszak, 1972; and Weizenbaum, 1972, 1976). The heterostatic theory suggests a different set of questions.

In examining the implications of the heterostatic theory for the AI paradigm, it should be noted that we will be concerned only with the long-term AI goal of realizing truly intelligent systems (systems that could be considered comparable to humans in intelligence). With regard to the short-term goal of accomplishing small practical increments in the intelligence of the conventional digital computer, AI researchers have demonstrated that they can do this. Their expectation, however, that these increments will eventually add up to a truly intelligent system or that a "critical mass" effect will occur at some point appears to have no basis. We will see below that a number of the assumptions underlying the AI paradigm appear questionable, relative to the AI researcher's long-term goal.

### 4.2.1  A Substrate for Intelligence

From the perspective of the heterostatic theory, a particular assumption of AI researchers emerges as being of crucial importance. It is a negative assumption that relates to a number of AI attributes. In Nilsson's (1974) survey of AI research, the assumption is stated as follows:

> ... knowledge about the structure and function of the neuron—or any other basic component of the brain—is irrelevant to the kind of understanding of intelligence that we are seeking. So long as these components can perform some very simple logical operations, then it doesn't really matter whether they are neurons, relays, vacuum-tubes, transistors, or whatever.

Implicit in this statement is the assumption that complex goal-seeking systems consist of simple non-goal-seeking components. Note that neurons are placed in a class with "relays, vacuum tubes, transistors, or whatever." Having unknowingly downgraded the neuron, AI researchers are then able to dismiss it as irrelevant. If the neuron is, in fact, a goal-seeking system in its own right, then Nilsson's (1974) introductory statement about AI needs to be considered in a new light. Nilsson states:

> The field of Artificial Intelligence (AI) has as its main tenet that there are indeed common processes that underlie thinking and perceiving, and furthermore that these processes can be understood and studied scientifically.

The present theory suggests that the heterostatic neuron represents the fundamental process underlying thinking and perceiving. If this is so, then the brain can no longer be envisioned as a collection of logic gates. Rather, it must be seen as an organized population of billions of goal-seeking "creatures," each "talking" to some thousands of others and each adapting its behavior in accordance with whether or not it is getting what it wants. Such a view of brain function calls into question certain aspects of the AI paradigm.

Artificial intelligence, as a part of theoretical psychology (Newell, 1970), assumes a top-down approach in which the mechanisms of intelligence are sought at high functional levels. Because the substrate can be shown to be of no consequence, *in principle* (we can use Turing machines, NOR gates, relays, vacuum tubes, etc.), AI researchers have gone on to assume that the substrate is of no consequence, *in practice*. But is that consistent with what biology teaches us?

Life has been evolving on this planet for approximately 3 billion years. Of that time, 90% was spent in evolving the neural substrate we share with the reptile. From the time of the reptile forward, it has been only a relatively short 300 million years until the emergence of humans. A question arises regarding the processes leading to intelligence. If the evolutionary process spent 90% of its time developing the neural substrate and the remaining 10% working out effective higher level mechanisms, why are artificial intelligence researchers attempting to do it the other way around? Admittedly, the evolutionary process could turn out, for a variety of reasons, to be a poor guide in choosing research strategies and allocating resources. However, the implications of the evolutionary process need to be considered, along with other reasons for questioning the AI researcher's strategy.

There has been a tendency among AI researchers to view the neuronal level as "primitive," but, perhaps, it would be better to think of this level as "detailed." It seems likely that an intelligent system will have to be built on a foundation that amounts to a highly detailed, immense *microscopic* knowledge base, a knowledge base that can be interfaced effectively with higher functional levels. A substrate consisting of goal-seeking adaptive network elements would seem to be well suited for such a purpose. Such a substrate appears to be consistent with the observation that humans, early on in life, develop microscopically "realistic" detailed perceptions of portions of their world that eventually are integrated into increasingly abstract, higher level views. In AI systems, the tendency has been to go quickly from the microscopically realistic to the macroscopically abstract at the front end in some kind of preprocessor. A scene is converted, for example, from a digitized image into some set of features so that then the "real" processing can begin. The preprocessing techniques differ fundamentally from the later more "intelligent" stages of information processing. One question to be considered is whether such a wide gulf between earlier and later stages of processing might be a fundamental obstacle to truly intelligent systems.

Consider how different the situation appears to be in such adaptive networks as nervous and social systems. As one moves up and down through the layers of a human social system, one observes that the "preprocessing" done at lower levels utilizes the same kinds of basic mechanisms that are employed at the higher levels for the more intelligent functions. For example, in the social "computations" involved in putting a man on the moon, from the lowest level functions involving, say, equipment fabrication to the highest level functions of NASA planning and mission execution, the techniques employed by the network elements (people) are fundamentally similar. This facilitates interfacing of functional layers in the hierarchy. There is no reason to believe it is different in nervous systems, although some unique preprocessing techniques are undoubtedly utilized on the sensory side.

### 4.2.2  The Role of Learning

Knowledge acquisition or learning is a central property of intelligence as we know it in living systems. It is, however, a process largely ignored in AI research. AI researchers have tended to factor intelligence into three components: knowledge acquisition, organization, and utilization. In living systems these three aspects of intelligence appear to be integral parts of a single process. This is also true for the heterostatic neuron. However, in AI research, where intelligence has been fractionated and the focus is on knowledge organization and use, learning has come to assume an unnatural role, as indicated by Nilsson's (1974) statement:

> ... we cannot have a program learn a fact before we know how to tell it that fact and before the program knows how to use that fact. We have been busy with telling and using facts. Learning them is still in the future. ...

Such prerequisite structuring of information before it can be learned is not the case for living systems, although it is true that prestructuring more nearly becomes a requirement as the information to be learned becomes more abstract.

The unnatural role of learning in AI systems can be related to the lack of a generalized goal. Highly specific goals do not lend themselves to the kind of general interaction with an environment that widely scoped learning probably requires. A generalized goal that can "drive" all of the activities of a system is needed. To obtain a generalized goal, the heterostatic theory suggests the following approach: translate all information for transmission into a pair of binary codes and then employ subsystems that seek to maximize the difference between the amounts of each of the two types of code being received. One code is to be sought by each subsystem and the other to be avoided. We hypothesized in earlier chapters that, in the case of the brain, the code that is sought employs excitation and that to be avoided employs inhibition. Such codes represent a generalization of the roles played by positive and negative feedback loops in conventional control systems. Perhaps greater coordination of subprograms and system generality can be achieved in AI systems with a similar approach. To some extent, this has been done in robotics research; for example, see Andreae (1964) and Doran (1968) where a robot's problems have been formulated in terms of variables similar to those of pleasure and pain (see review by Ernst, 1970).

Among AI researchers, the need for learning mechanisms is being increasingly felt. Nilsson (1974) states:

> Today, the knowledge in a program must be put in "by hand" by the programmer although there are beginning attempts at getting programs to acquire knowledge through on-line interaction with skilled humans. To build really large knowledgeable systems, we will have to educate existing programs rather than attempt the almost impossible feat of giving birth to already competent ones.

To date, AI researchers have employed both procedural and declarative representations for knowledge. Learning, if it is based on a generalized goal-seeking mechanism, will by the very nature of the mechanism favor procedural representations. Also, a change in attitude will be required on the part of those who structure the environments for and train such systems. In the case of a system possessing a generalized goal, it will become important to ask not only what the machine can do for us, but also what we can do for the machine.

Regarding learning, perhaps one further comment is in order. The training of adaptive networks has become associated with the dreary repetition of some specific set of stimuli until the correct responses are learned. However, when truly intelligent systems are developed, it probably will not work that way. Just as in the case of living systems, the repetition will be accomplished by immersing the system in its environment for a substantial period, until it becomes firmly embedded through a large number of positively and negatively reinforcing feedback loops. The system will then emerge with the kind of microscopic knowledge base that can support the more macroscopic mechanisms associated with intelligence.

### 4.2.3  Knowledge Bases

AI researchers started out a couple of decades ago seeking a psychologically oriented version of intelligence. Understandably, they wanted to be spared the pain of wrestling with the kinds of neurophysiologically oriented details that adaptive network researchers seemed to be hung up on. AI researchers felt that they were going directly to the solution. It was a worthwhile attempt but at this point we know that it did not work. The General Problem Solvers, theorem provers, question answerers and other similar kinds of systems of the early 1960s were found to lack generality and to lack power.

When this became clear, AI researchers stood back and reexamined the problem. They concluded that a somewhat less abstract approach would be required. It was decided that what was needed for a successful system was an immense knowledge base. Thus, more recent AI research has been concerned with the questions of how to organize and utilize immense knowledge bases. (As noted above, AI researchers generally assume that the problem of knowledge *acquisition* can be decoupled from the problems of organization and utilization.) The question now is whether substantially increased intelligence will come with larger knowledge bases? Surely some gains are being made, but unless the nature of these knowledge bases changes drastically, it seems unlikely that truly intelligent systems will result. The very notion of a "knowledge base" suggests a passive approach to learning and memory, an approach rooted in von Neumann's design for the conventional digital computer. An implication of the heterostatic theory is that much more active (and microscopically detailed) knowledge bases will be required than the relatively passive (and macroscopically oriented) knowledge bases currently being pursued in AI research.

It is true that the procedural nets, semantic nets, inference nets, and frame theories currently being investigated by AI researchers (see, for example, Bobrow and Collins, 1975; or Minsky, 1975) all suggest movement in the direction of an adaptive networklike formulation, albeit at a macroscopic level. However, the character of these knowledge bases is still very much determined by the AI researcher's orientation toward conventional digital computers. What would seem to be required is much more movement in the direction of what we might call non-von Neumann approaches.

Such movement appears to be occurring in the work of Minsky and Papert (1977) . They have begun to invoke nervous system/social system parallels in their work on a theory they call "the society of minds." Minsky and Papert are developing a psychologically oriented theory based on hierarchies of local agents they term "doers," "critics," and "censors." Thus, the possibility arises of an ultimate and fruitful convergence of adaptive network and artificial intelligence research with adaptive network researchers approaching the problem from the bottom up and artificial intelligence researchers approaching it from the top down.

## 4.2.4  The Nature of Intelligence

The character of artificial intelligence, as it has developed to date, appears to differ in fundamental ways from the character of natural intelligence. In contrast to the relatively passive and detached view of intelligence implicit in AI-oriented knowledge bases, Arbib (1972, 1975b) has suggested that intelligence in living systems is active and embedded. Arbib's formulation in terms of "action-oriented" computations emphasizes the goal-seeking nature of natural intelligence. In contrast, AI systems often appear to possess more of an open-loop than a closed-loop (goal-seeking) character.

Furthermore, to the extent that AI systems are goal-seeking, the nature of the goals pursued is quite different from those pursued by living systems. AI systems generally pursue what may be termed *external goals*. That is to say, the system's efforts are directed at altering the state of the environment in some way. The AI formulation tends to be in terms of relatively fixed (but flexible) internal procedures dealing with a variable external environment. Living systems, on the other hand, appear to be better understood in terms of the pursuit of *internal goals* through variable (adaptive) internal procedures operating on a relatively fixed external environment.

Whether one views intelligent systems and their environments as changing or unchanging and whether one views goals as internal or external is, in the most fundamental sense, however, to make arbitrary distinctions. This is because of the kind of "yin yang" relationship that holds between an intelligent system and its environment. For example, whether one views the state of a game of chess as changing or the nature of the game as unchanging and whether one views the AI system playing the game as pursuing the internal goal of a "win" state or the external goal of checkmate is, in the final analysis, to make distinctions that simply reflect different viewpoints. That is not to say that such distinctions are unimportant. In formulating theories of intelligent systems, there is a need to consider, for example, whether it will be more productive to think in terms of internal or external goals.

There is another way in which the AI researcher's perception of intelligence appears not to be consonant with the nature of the phenomenon in living systems. (Actually, the comment that follows applies more to the first decade of AI research than to the second.) In living systems, intelligence frequently is not intelligent, at least not in the intellectual sense in which AI researchers have sometimes viewed the phenomenon. Rather, intelligence in living systems is frequently simply *effective*. There would appear to be much that is of a "brute force" nature in the everyday information processing of intelligent organisms. Immense numbers of stimuli are mapped, in a more or less straightforward fashion, into immense numbers of responses, such that the organism gets along in a day-to-day pleasure seeking and survival sense. Even for the most intelligent humans, the more intellectual forms of activity are difficult. For example, correct generalizations are not easily arrived at and really new ideas in research are an absolute rarity. Thus, one wonders if the association of intelligence with higher level information processing has, perhaps, left the AI researcher with too narrow and elevated a view of the phenomenon. In the near term, would a more modest view yield more productive theories?

## 4.2.5   Implications of the Mind-Body Problem

The problem of developing intelligent hardware may have two aspects: (1) developing an inherently self-organizing substrate and (2) developing an effective higher level organization utilizing the substrate. AI researchers may be prematurely addressing the second question first.

AI researchers have devoted much of their attention to information processing mechanisms of the kind that, in people, occur at a conscious (or near-conscious) level. That is to say, AI researchers tend to investigate those mechanisms that occur at the level of the mind. But what fraction of the total information processing accomplished within the human brain is conscious (and therefore AI-like) and how much is of a more elementary nature corresponding to subconscious and unconscious processes? If the mind corresponds to the midbrain and thalamic reticular formation, as was hypothesized in Chapter 4, it follows that conscious information processing constitutes, perhaps, only 1/1000 of all of the information processing occurring in the human brain. When conscious information processing is viewed in this way, it can be seen that AI researchers have been investigating the "tip of the iceberg." It is as though AI researchers have been attempting to construct the top floor of a 1000-story building. The promised view is, indeed, exciting, but without the first 999 floors, the actual view will necessarily be disappointing.

In one sense, AI research has focused almost exclusively on the functions of the mind, or what we might term the conscious command and control center aspects of intelligence. In another sense, AI researchers have been able to largely ignore the question of command and control. This has been possible because AI systems have not been highly parallel and decentralized in their operation. Only when one "deploys" a large number of semi-autonomous adaptive components does the command and control function become important. Then, one must ask, where does ultimate control reside? Is the control function just handed off from one part of the system to another as the environmental inputs drive the system into various states? Something like this would seem to be the view of those who believe that the seat of consciousness is partly or totally in the neocortex. For AI researchers, the question will become more important if their systems become highly parallel and decentralized.

The AI researcher's tendency to focus on conscious information processing may be viewed in another way. Such high level processing is quite clearly a linguistically oriented function. However, the real language of intelligence is probably not linguistic, but rather sublinguistic. AI research is focused on higher order language realizations of intelligence but, for truly intelligent hardware, we may have to develop an adequate "machine language" first. In the case of the living brain, a remarkably effective machine language, based on the excitatory and inhibitory pulse trains that are formed out of neuronal action potentials, has already been developed. Much that is fundamental to intelligence in any form probably occurs at this level.

### 4.2.6 Summary

Table 2 summarizes the differences that have been suggested between the AI researcher's view of intelligence, on the one

**TABLE 2.** Adaptive Networks and Artificial Intelligence—Alternative Research Strategies

| Contrasts | Approaches | |
| --- | --- | --- |
| | Adaptive networks | Artificial intelligence |
| Functional level<br>Biological analog | Microscopic<br>Neurophysiology | Macroscopic<br>Psychology |
| Epistemological assumption | Knowledge acquisition, representation, and utilization are nonseparable aspects of a single integral process. | Knowledge acquisition, representation, and utilization are separable processes for research purposes. Acquisition (learning) can be addressed at some future time. |
| Local assumption<br>Global assumption | Neuron = Goal-seeking component<br>Mind = Upper brain stem (localized command-and-control) | Neuron = Non-goal-seeking component<br>Mind = ? (Position not established but prevailing tendency today is to view the mind as corresponding to the cortex or the whole brain, implying distributed command-and-control) |
| Nature of substrate | Decentralized, parallel, pervasively adaptive | Centralized, serial, nonadaptive (conventional digital computer) |
| Nature of knowledge base | Immense, microscopic, realistic | Limited, macroscopic, abstract |
| Nature of goals<br>Nature of system | Generalized and internal<br>Active and embedded | Specialized and external<br>Passive and detached |
| Likely payoff of research | Inherently self-organizing substrate for intelligent information processing systems | "Psychology" of conventional digital computers |

hand, and the proposed adaptive network view, on the other. The two approaches to intelligence are contrasted with respect to a number of fundamental assumptions. While it is clear that AI research must continue if we are to establish the limits of the digital computer's capabilities, there appears to be no basis for expecting that this research can ever yield systems of an intelligence comparable to that of humans. AI research, in employing a centralized, serial, nonadaptive substrate (a conventional digital computer) appears to be 180 degrees out of phase with the one architecture that is known to work, namely that of the living brain. For highly intelligent systems, it seems likely that research into decentralized, parallel, pervasively adaptive networks will be required, based on substrates of goal-seeking components.

## 4.3  A BASIC BUILDING BLOCK

One of the objectives of adaptive network research has been to obtain an element that could serve as a fundamental building block for the construction of a wide variety of adaptive systems. At one point, it was thought that the variable-weighted linear threshold element, in conjunction with the algorithmic adaptive procedure provided by the perceptron convergence theorem, was such an element. The present theory offers a new candidate element: the heterostat. The *elementary heterostat* (one that cannot be reduced further to component heterostatic subsystems) is a device that appears to meet the requirements. Such a claim is based on the conclusion that it is the heterostatic nature of neurons that is responsible for the information processing capabilities of nervous systems.

An elementary heterostat derives its power from the special way in which it utilizes feedback information. In the case of positive feedback (e.g., excitation delivered to a neuron), not only does the input enhance the output, but also *the input enhances the effectiveness of recently active positive feedback loops*. In the case of negative feedback (e.g., inhibition delivered to a neuron), not only does the input diminish the output, but also *the input enhances the effectiveness of recently active inhibitory feedback loops*. In this way, the heterostat not only accomplishes short-term, but also long-term, modifications in its behavior, thus encoding causal relations and providing a basis for intelligence.

## 4.4 FUTURE RESEARCH

Understanding of heterostatic networks will have to be sought primarily through experimental studies of synthesized and biological networks. More rigorous analytical approaches are generally not possible with currently available mathematical techniques (and it is not clear that this situation will ever improve much for complex networks).

Initially, in the study of small synthesized networks of elementary heterostats, the dynamics of the systems may be more readily analyzed if the networks do not interact with an environment, other than the environment provided by other elements in the network. This simplification will permit attention to be focused on the interactions among network elements. Such isolated systems might provide adequate models for neural and social networks where all relevant inputs originate in other heterostats. The model will not be satisfactory for any system in which some of the inputs originate in the environment within which the system is embedded.

Beyond the study of such isolated systems, the more general problem will be that of establishing the relationship between a heterostatic system's structure and the system's effectiveness in eliciting positive stimuli from an environment while avoiding negative stimuli. (In this discussion, "positive" and "negative" will refer to the categories that, in the special case of living systems, might be described as pleasurable and painful, appetitive and aversive, depolarizing and hyperpolarizing, or excitatory and inhibitory.) The question of how a heterostatic system and an environment should be structured if it is desired that the network learn to solve a particular problem will be of immediate practical interest. In all of this work, it will be important to develop methods for classifying the structures of environments and of heterostatic systems, so that a wide variety of possibilities can be studied efficiently.

The sequence of developments during future experimental

studies will necessarily parallel, to some extent, the developments that must have occurred during the evolution of nervous systems. Initially, simple networks of elementary heterostats can be studied interacting with simple environments, perhaps paralleling the evolutionary phase during which simple multicellular organisms interacted with the simple environment of the sea. It will be necessary to provide the synthesized networks with sensory transducers that can convert environmental stimuli into positive and negative inputs. Motor transducers will convert positive and negative outputs into actions affecting the environment. As it becomes possible to synthesize larger and more complex systems, a variety of subsystems will "evolve," including specialized command and control centers, reinforcement centers that will impose a global type of pressure on the elements so that they will adapt in particular directions, drive centers that will supply innate knowledge, and memory centers that will permit the more effective utilization of past experience.

# Chapter 5
# concluding remarks

It is difficult if not impossible to draw a line separating the regulatory behavior of lower organisms from the so-called intelligent behavior of higher ones; the one grades insensibly into the other. From the lowest organisms up to man behavior is essentially regulatory in character, and what we call intelligence in higher animals is a direct outgrowth of the same laws that give behavior its regulatory character in the Protozoa.

*H. S. Jennings (1906)*

In attempting to understand the elements out of which mental phenomena are compounded, it is of the greatest importance to remember that from the protozoa to man there is nowhere a very wide gap either in structure or in behavior. From this fact it is a highly probable inference that there is also nowhere a very wide mental gap.

*B. Russell (1921)*

To declare that, of the component cells that go to make us up, each one is an individual self-centered life is no mere phrase. It is not a mere convenience for descriptive purposes. The cell as a component of the body is not only a visibly demarcated unit but a unit-life centered on itself. It leads its own life ... The cell is a unit-life, and our life which in its turn is a unitary life consists utterly of cell-lives.

*C. S. Sherrington (1941)*

If neurons are heterostats and, furthermore, if organized collections of neurons (nervous systems) are heterostats, then it seems reasonable to consider that organized collections of nervous systems (social systems) may also be heterostats. The observed behavior of social systems would seem to support such a hypothesis. Actually, the list can be broadened. It is anticipated that the class of heterostatic systems includes neurons, assemblies of neurons, whole nervous systems, families, neighborhoods, cities, regions, and nations.

A system is a heterostat if it is organized in such a way that it seeks to maximize a specific internal variable. In the case of social systems, that variable is hypothesized to be the total amount of pleasure being experienced by the system's members (pain, in this context, constitutes negative pleasure). Actually, to suggest that a nervous system or a social system functions as a single, integrated heterostat is to simplify the matter. It is usually the case that some part of the system occupies a position of control and it, functioning as a heterostat, imposes constraints on the remaining subsystems. These subsystems, in turn, may also function as heterostats, but in doing so, they will be subject to the imposed constraints from the controlling subsystem. Thus, in general, it is hypothesized that nervous systems and social systems are organized as collections of interacting heterostatic subsystems. Furthermore, each subsystem may consist of a collection of heterostatic "subsubsystems" where one is in control and the remainder are subject to imposed constraints. In this way, the regression may continue down to some fundamental level.

To consider an example, it was hypothesized earlier that the MTRF is the controlling subsystem of the brain and, furthermore, that it is a heterostat. That is to say, it seeks to maximize the amount of polarization being experienced by MTRF neurons; it does not seek to maximize the amount of polarization being experienced by all neurons within the brain. Thus, the brain is hypothesized to be a heterostatic system in which the controlling subsystem is a heterostat, as are the controlled subsystems. In general, we may define a heterostatic system as one in which either (a) the heterostatic variable $\mu$ is defined with respect to all of the subsystems taken collectively, that is, the system functions as a single, integrated heterostat, or (b) $\mu$ is defined with respect to the controlling subsystem, as in the case of the MTRF of the brain. The first type of system will be termed an *integrated heterostat*; the second type will be termed a *limited heterostat*. An integrated heterostat is organized such that whenever $\mu$ for each of the subsystems is maximized, so is $\mu$ for the system as a whole. In the case of social systems, this is, perhaps, the necessary and sufficient condition for the achievement of a perfect democracy. Alternatively, a society that assumes the form of a dictatorship provides an example of a limited heterostat.

The brain appears to be organized as a limited heterostat. Does this evolutionary outcome imply that a limited heterostat represents a more stable form of organization than the integrated heterostat? Such may be the implication at the neural level, but an extrapolation to the societal level may not be valid. However, it is a question that appears to be relevant if one desires to compare, for example, the life expectancies of democracies and dictatorships.

It can be seen that the present theory offers the possibility of a unified systems approach to the study of adaptive networks, whether they be of the neural, social, or man-made variety. It should be possible to construct a single heterostatic model of an adaptive network such that the model would simultaneously possess relevance for the neurophysiologist, psychologist, sociologist, and cybernetician. This model would consist, essentially, of a set of nested heterostatic subsystems. Each subsystem would receive two types of input, one type to be sought, the other to be avoided, these inputs being variously described as excitatory or inhibitory, appetitive or aversive, pleasurable or painful, and, perhaps, positive or negative, depending on the particular application. A generalized version of the neuronal process of heterostatic adaptation would provide the maximization mechanism for each subsystem.

## 5.1 COMPARING SOCIAL SYSTEMS WITH NERVOUS SYSTEMS

If indeed brains and societies are fundamentally similar kinds of systems, then a comparison of their behavioral characteristics should be instructive. For a start, we might consider that brains exhibit three properties that have been of substantial interest: brain functions are distributed, redundant, and (sometimes) recoverable after extensive damage. Societal functions possess these three properties also. The knowledge and skills contained within a society are, in general, not highly localized. Furthermore, just as it may be normal for neurons to die each day while the nervous system, utilizing its redundant structure, continues to function, so, too, does the continual loss of members go on in a society without rendering the system unworkable.

With either brains or societies, however, if the damage to the system is extensive so that redundancy of function cannot adequately compensate, then a process of adaptation will in some cases permit the function to be recovered. In the case of the brain, it was hypothesized that this recovery occurs because the surviving neurons are subjected to a new set of input conditions and, thus, they modify their transmittances so as to once more tend to maximize the amount of polarization they are experiencing. It was suggested that these transmittance changes and the recovery of function are one and the same process. The mechanism would appear to be the same within a society. When a substantial portion of a social system is destroyed due to a natural disaster or due to war, the surviving members can be seen to respond to their new input conditions in such a way as to once more tend to maximize the amount of pleasure they are experiencing. Often, to accomplish this, they must learn to perform the function previously accomplished by that portion of the society that has been destroyed. We have marveled at the brain's ability to recover functions after extensive damage. The same process, occurring within a society, produces less awe because the mechanism is more apparent. We can generalize here. Perhaps one of the best ways to gain an appreciation of how neurons may interact is to observe how people interact within the various social systems of which they are a part. If one adopts this viewpoint, the properties of brains become less mysterious. (For anyone interested in nervous system/social system analogies, Crane's (1978) exploration of possible parallels is recommended.)

It may be noted that distributed functions, redundancy, and recoverability of function through adaptation are not always adequate protection either in the case of brains or societies. Certain heterostatic subsystems are of critical importance and their loss results in great and permanent damage to the total organization. The MTRF of the brain and the capital cities of some nations serve as examples of such subsystems.

## 5.2 RESTRUCTURING SOCIAL SYSTEMS

If one observes a human social system for an extended period, it becomes clear that fundamental to such an adaptive network are the transactions carried out at a local level among the goal-seeking adaptive components, which is to say, among its people. The transactions involve large numbers of positively and negatively reinforcing feedback loops that appear to be basic to the human substrate on which a successful society is built. When many of these local feedback loops are cut in favor of more centralized mechanisms, the result is usually reduced efficiency.

In the context of the present theory, it is concluded that neurons do not exist for the sake of nervous systems, nor people for the sake of social systems. People will generally do what is best for their society when it coincides with what is best for themselves. Therefore, a society can achieve a particular result most efficiently if it assumes a structure that provides for a coincidence of the interests of the individual and the society.

In what ways can present societies be restructured in order to enable them to better meet the needs of their members? Some possible answers to this question are suggested by observing ways in which societies and brains differ in their organizational structures.

First of all, governments have a tendency to make their decisions at the top and to execute them at the bottom. Nervous systems, on the other hand, appear to make increasingly detailed decisions all along the line, as one moves from the upper to the lower levels in the hierarchy. In addition to establishing general goals, the upper control levels in the brain appear to regulate by delivering reward or punishment *based on the results obtained*, not based on whether a detailed plan of action passed down from above was followed. Is the evolutionary process suggesting to us that a high degree of decentralization is the most effective organizational structure for a society? One cannot be sure of such an extrapolation, of course, but we should carefully consider advice that has survived millions of years of selection.

Second, in reinforcing neuronal behavior, brains appear to employ a mix of reward and punishment. On the other hand, governments tend to employ only punishment. The services provided in return for taxes do not constitute positive reinforcement because our receipt of them is not, in general, contingent upon our behavior. Essentially, the only behavior-contingent response is the punishment received when one has broken a law. In contrast, note that many private organizations do employ a mix of rewards and punishments and the result appears to be more effective organizations. Promotions, pay raises, profit sharing, recognition, prestige, and power are highly effective positive reinforcers. The denial of these rewards, or even more extreme, the loss of one's job, provides effective punishment. Such a balanced set of reinforcers does not confront the citizen in his relationship to his government. Rather, the name of the game for many simply becomes that of avoiding punishment. Skinner (1971) has recognized, perhaps better than anyone else, the need for us to rectify this situation by building social institutions that implement a more suitable variety of reinforcers.

Finally, concerning the subject of international cooperation, the present theory suggests what many already know. A nation will not willingly surrender power to an international organization unless a point is reached where it is in the nation's best interest to do so. The nature of heterostats is such that they do not cooperate as parts of larger heterostatic systems unless they have more reward than punishment to gain by doing so. Such was the case for neurons, and heterostatic brains emerged. Such was the case for people, and heterostatic societies emerged. Will such be the case for nations and will, finally, a single heterostatic earth-society eventually emerge? The hazards of gross ecological imbalance and the prospects for nuclear annihilation are potential negative reinforcers of great power. The benefits of cooperation could be many.

## 5.3 SUMMARY

At the fundamental level of the cell, and, consequently, at higher levels, life in its more intelligent forms is seen to be a process aimed at achieving a maximal condition. With this as its goal, advanced living systems utilize positive and negative feedback loops in such a way as to accomplish long-term adaptation as well as the regulation of immediate behavior.

Both positive and negative feedback are essential to life's processes. However, it is positive feedback that is the dominant force—it provides the "spark of life." It is the effects of positive feedback that account for observations such as Sherrington's (1941):

> "Life has an itch to live." This itch is universal with it. Under the microscope it gives us tiny lives hurrying hither, thither, feeding. Driven, each says almost as clearly as if it spoke, by "urge-to-life." The one key phrase to the whole bustling scene seems "urge-to-live."

> If, from the microscope, we turn to look at the busy street, with its individuals hurrying hither and thither, hastening to earn, entering restaurants, is there no resemblance to that other, the microscopic scene? What phrase again sums it up? "Urge-to-live." And here, becuase we know it in ourselves, we can read securely into that urge, as of it and with it, an element "zeal-to-live," "zest-to-live." The physico-chemical has here its mental adjunct. Life's zest to live as outcome of life's tendency to increase in bulk. Long the stretch of distance between that microscopic population and this human one. Yet if a form of mind there be in that microscopic population, though as a germ so remote that no word of ours can duly fit it, is it not probable that that mind is "zest-to-live" in germ?

The evolutionary process has established an equivalence between that which has survival value and that which is a source of pleasure. Thus, living systems, in pursuing heterostasis, participate in three broad categories of actions:

1. Self-preserving behavior (maintenance of homeostasis)
2. Species-preserving behavior (reproduction)

3. Stimulation-preserving behavior (knowledge acquisition and play)

Recognition that these categories represent *sub*goals, pursued only as means to an end (heterostasis), renders certain aspects of human behavior more understandable. We can see why it is that people go on making love *and* war while researching both subjects. Concerning stimulation-preserving behavior, it is seen that it is not the sometimes postulated "need to understand" that drives humans to explore their universe; rather, it is the need for stimulation.

In conclusion, it is seen that complex forms of behavior in living systems derive not from complex underlying mechanisms but from the combinatorics of billions of interacting subunits and from the complexity of environments. A simple perspective emerges. Neurons, nervous systems, and nations are heterostats.

# references

Adametz, J. H. (1959) Rate of recovery of functioning in cats with rostral reticular lesions. *J. Neurosurg.* 16:85-97.

Andersen, P., Eccles, J. C., and Voorhoeve, P. E. (1963) Inhibitory synapses of somas of purkinje cells in the cerebellum. *Nature* 194:740-741.

Andersen, P., Eccles, J. C., and Lyning, Y. (1963) Recurrent inhibition in the hippocampus with identification of the inhibitory cell and its synapses. *Nature* 198:541-542.

Andreae, J. H. (1964) STELLA: a scheme for a learning machine. *Proc. 2nd IFAC Congress.* Butterworth, London, pp. 497-502.

Arbib, M. A. (1972) *The metaphorical brain*. Wiley-Interscience, New York.

Arbib, M. A. (1975a) From automata theory to brain theory. *Int. J. Man-Mach. Stud.* 7:279-295.

Arbib, M. A. (1975b) Artificial intelligence and brain theory: Unities and diversities. *Ann. Biomed. Eng.* 3:238-274.

Aristotle (384-322 B. C.) *Nicomachean ethics*. Loeb Classical Library, Harvard University, 1939, p. 31.

Ashby, W. (1952, 1960) *Design for a brain*. Wiley, New York.

Bernard, C. (1859) Lecons sur les proprietes physiologigues et les alterations pathologigues des liquides de l'organisme. *Balliere 1*, Paris, France.

Bindman, L. J., Lippold, O. C. J., and Redfearn, J. W. T. (1964) The action of brief polarizing currents on the cerebral cortex of the rat (1) during current flow and (2) in the production of long-lasting aftereffects. *J. Physiol.* 172:369-382.

Blackstad, T. W., and Flood, P. R. (1963) Ultrastructure and hippocampal axosomatic synapses. *Nature* 198:542-543.

Bobrow, D. G., and Collins, A. (1975) *Representation and understanding: Studies in cognitive science*. Academic Press, New York.

Boden, M. (1977) *Artificial intelligence and natural man*. Basic Books, New York.

Bogen, J. E. (1969) The other side of the brain II: An appositional mind. *Bull. Los Angeles Neuro. Soc.* 34:135-162.

Brain, A., Forsen, G., Hall, D., and Rosen, C. (1963) A large, self-contained learning machine. *1963 WESCON Paper 6.1* VII (part 4).

Bures, J., and Buresova, O. (1965) Discussion. Plasticity at the single neuron level. *Proc. Int. Union Physiol. Sci.* (Twenty-third International Congress at Tokyo) 4:359-364.

Bures, J., and Buresova, O. (1967) Spreading depression and corticosubcortical interrelations in the mechanism of conditioned reflexes. *Progr. Brain Res.* 22:378-387.

Bures, J., and Buresova, O. (1970) Plasticity in single neurons and neural populations. In *Short-term changes in neural activity and behavior* (eds. G. Horn and R. A. Hinde). Cambridge University Press, New York, pp. 363-403.

Burns, B. D. (1968) *The uncertain nervous system*. Edward Arnold Ltd., London.

Campbell, H. J. (1973) *The pleasure areas*. Delacorte, New York.

Cannon, W. B. (1929) Organization for physiological homeostasis. *Physiol. Rev.* 9:399-431.

Chow, K. L. (1961) Brain functions. *Ann. Rev. Psych.* 12:281-310.

Crane, H. D. (1978) *Beyond the seventh synapse: The neural marketplace of the mind*. Research Memorandum, SRI International, Menlo Park, California.

Cunningham, M. (1972) *Intelligence: Its organization and development*. Academic Press, New York.

Delafresnaye, J. F. (1954) *Brain mechanisms and consciousness*. Thomas, Springfield, Illinois.

Delgado, J. M. R., Roberts, W. W., and Miller, N. E. (1954) Learning motivated by electrical stimulation of the brain. *Amer. J. Physiol.* 179:587.

Dement, W. (1960) The effect of dream deprivation. *Science* 131:1705.

Dement, W., and Kleitman, N. (1957) *J. Exper. Psycho.* 53:339.

Doran, J. E. (1968) Experiments with a pleasure-seeking automaton. *Machine Intelligence 3* (ed. Donald Michie). Elsevier, New York, pp. 195-216.

Dreyfus, H. L. (1965) *Alchemy and artificial intelligence*. RAND Corporation Paper P3244 (AD 625 719).

Dreyfus, H. L. (1972) *What computers can't do*. Harper and Row, New York.

Eccles, J. C. (1953) *The neurophysiological basis of mind: The principles of neurophysiology*. Clarendon Press, Oxford.

Eccles, J. C. (1964) *The physiology of synapses*. Academic Press, New York.

Eccles, J. C. (1966) Conscious experience and memory. In *Brain and conscious experience* (ed. J. C. Eccles). Springer-Verlag, New York, pp. 314–344.

Eccles, J. C. (1969a) *The inhibitory pathways of the central nervous system*. Liverpool University Press, Liverpool, p. 135.

Eccles, J. C. (1969b) Excitatory and inhibitory mechanisms in brain. In *Basic mechanisms of the epilepsies* (eds. H. H. Jasper, A. A. Ward, Jr., and A. Pope). Little, Brown and Company, Boston, pp. 229–252.

Eccles, J. C., Ito, M., and Szentagothai, J. (1969) *The cerebellum as a neuronal machine*. Springer-Verlag, New York, p. 335.

Eddington, A. (1958) *The nature of the physical world*. University of Michigan Press, Ann Arbor.

Ernst, H. A. (1970) *Computer-Controlled Robots*. IBM Research Report RC 2781 (No. 13043).

Ettlinger, G., Blakemore, C. B., Milner, A. D., and Wilson, J. (1974) Agenesis of corpus callosum: A further behavioral investigation. *Brain* 97 (Pt. 2): 225–234.

Farley, B. G., and Clark, W. A. (1954) Simulation of a self organizing system by a digital computer. *IRE Trans. Inf. Theory* PGIT-4:76–84.

Feigenbaum, E. A., and Feldman, J. (1963) *Computers and thought*. McGraw-Hill, New York.

Feigl, H. (1958) The 'mental' and the 'physical.' In *Minnesota studies in the philosophy of science*. Vol. II (eds. H. Feigl, M. Scriven, and G. Maxwell). University of Minnesota Press, Minneapolis, pp. 370–497.

Feigl, H. (1960) Mind-body, *not* a pseudoproblem. In *Dimensions of mind*, (ed. Sidney Hook). Collier Books, New York, pp. 33–44.

Fessard, A. E. (1954) Mechanisms of nervous integration and conscious experience, *Brain mechanisms and consciousness* (eds. E. O. Adrian, F. Bremer, and H. Jasper). Thomas, Springfield, Illinois, pp. 200–236.

Finley, M. (1967) *An experimental study of the formation and development of Hebbian cell-assemblies by means of a neural network simulation*. Technical Report, Department of Communications Sciences, University of Michigan, Ann Arbor.

Freud, S. (1895, 1964) Untitled paper. In *Standard edition of the complete psychological works of Freud* Vol. I (ed. James Strachey). Macmillan, New York, pp. 281–387.

Fuxe, K. (1965) *Acta Physiol. Scand.* 64 (Suppl. 247):37–84.

Gamba, A., Bamberini, L., Palmieri, G., and Sanna, R. (1961) Further experiments with PAPA, *Nuovo Cimento Suppl.* 20 (No. 2):221–231.

Gazzaniga, M. S. (1967) The split brain in man. *Sci. Am.* 217 (2):24–29.

Gazzaniga, M. S. (1970) *The bisected brain*. Appleton-Century-Crofts, New York.

Gazzaniga, M. S. (1972) One brain-two minds? *Am. Sci.* 60:311-317.

Gazzaniga, M. S., LeDoux, J. E. (1978) *The integrated mind.* Plenum, New York

Gerbrandt, L. K., Skrebitsky, V. G., Buresova, O., and Bures, J. (1968) Plastic changes of unit activity induced by tactile stimuli followed by electrical stimulation of single hippocampal and reticular neurons. *Neuropsychologia* 6:3-10.

Globus, G. G. (1976) Mind, structure and contradiction. In *Consciousness and the brain: A scientific and philosophical inquiry* (eds. G. Globus, G. Maxwell, and I. Savodnik). Plenum Press, New York, pp. 271-293.

Goddard, G. V. (1967) Development of epileptic seizures through brain stimulation at low intensity. *Nature* 214:1020.

Good, I. J. (1965) Speculations concerning the first ultraintelligent machine. *Adv. Comput.* 6:31-88.

Griffin, J. P. (1970) Neurophysiological studies into habituation. *Short-term changes in neural activity and behavior* (eds. G. Horn and R. A. Hinde). Cambridge University Press, New York, pp. 141-179.

Griffith, V. V. (1962) *A mathematical model of the plastic neuron.* Goodyear Aircraft Corporation, Akron, Ohio, Rept. No. GER-10589.

Griffith, V. V. (1963) A model of the plastic neuron. *IEEE Trans. Military Electron.* MIL-7:243-253.

Guerrero-Figueroa, R., Barros, A., Heath, R. G., and Gonzalez, G. (1964) Experimental subcortical epileptiform focus. *Epilepsia* 5:112.

Gurowitz, E. M. (1969) *The molecular basis of memory.* Prentice-Hall, Englewood Cliffs, New Jersey.

Hartmann, E. L. (1966) *Int. J. Psychiatry.* 2:11.

Hartmann, E. L. (1973) *The functions of sleep.* Yale University Press, New Haven, Connecticut.

Haug, H. (1972) Stereological methods in the analysis of neuronal parameters in the central nervous system. *J. Microscopy* 95 (Pt. 1):165-180.

Heath, R. B., and Mickel, W. A. (1960) Evaluation of seven years' experience with depth electrode studies in human patients. In *Electrical studies on the unanesthetized brain* (eds. E. R. Ramey and D. S. O'Doherty). Harper, New York.

Hebb, D. O. (1949) *Organization of behavior.* Wiley, New York.

Hilgard, E. R. (1969) Pain as a puzzle for psychology and physiology. *Am. Psychol.* 24:103-113.

Hillarp, N. A., Fuxe, K., and Dahlstrom, A. (1966) Demonstration and mapping of central neurons containing dopamine, noradrenaline, and 5-hydroxytryptamine and their reactions to psychopharmaca. *Pharmacol. Rev.* 18:727.

Hoebel, B. G. (1971) Feeding: Neural control of intake. *Ann. Rev. Physiol.* 33:533–568.

Holmgren, B., and Frenk, S. (1961) Inhibitory phenomena and 'habituation' at the neuronal level. *Nature* 192:1294–1295.

Horn, G., and Hinde, R. A. (1970) *Short-term changes in neural activity and behavior.* Cambridge University Press, New York.

Hubel, D. H., and Wiesel, T. N. (1965) Binocular interaction in striate cortex of kittens reared with artificial squint. *J. Neurophysiol.* 28:1040–1072.

Hull, C. L. (1943) *Principles of behavior.* Appleton-Century-Crofts, New York.

Jaynes, J. (1977) *The origin of consciousness in the breakdown of the bicameral mind.* Houghton Mifflin, Boston.

Jennings, H. S. (1906) *Behavior of the lower organisms.* Columbia University Press, New York, p. 335.

John, E. R. (1976) A model of consciousness. In *Consciousness and self-regulation* Vol. 1 (eds., G. E. Schwartz, and D. Shapairo). Plenum Press, New York, pp. 1–50.

Jung, R. (1953) Allgemeine neurophysiologie. In *Handbuch der Inneren Medizin.* Springer, Berlin, pp. 1–181.

Kandel, E. R. (1974) An invertebrate system for the cellular analysis of simple behaviors and their modifications. In *The neurosciences: Third study program* (eds. F. O. Schmitt, and F. G. Warden). M.I.T. Press, Cambridge, Mass.

Kaylor, D. J. (1964) *A mathematical model of a two-layer network of threshold elements.* Rome Air Development Center Technical Documentary Report, RADC-TDR-63-534.

Kilmer, W. L. (1975) Biology of decisionary and learning mechanisms in mammalian CA3-hippocampus (a review). *Int. J. Man-Mach. Stud.* 7:413.

Kilmer, W. L., McCulloch, W. S., and Blum, H. (1967) *Some mechanisms for a theory of the reticular formation.* Final Scientific Report: AF-AFOSR-1023-66.

Kilmer, W. L., McCulloch, W. S., and Blum, J. (1969) A model of the vertebrate central command system. *Int. J. Man-Mach. Stud.* 1:279.

Kling, J. W., and Stevenson, J. G. (1970) Habituation and extinction. In *Short-term changes in neural activity and behavior* (eds. G. Horn and R. A. Hinde). Cambridge University Press, New York, pp. 41–61.

Klopf, A. H. (1971) *Design and simulation of locally and globally adaptive multilevel networks.* Ph.D. Thesis, University of Illinois at the Medical Center, Chicago (available from University Microfilms, Ann Arbor, Michigan).

Klopf, A. H. (1972) *Brain function and adaptive systems—A heterostatic theory.* Air Force Cambridge Research Laboratories Special Report No. 133 (AFCRL-72-0164), L. G. Hanscom Field, Bedford, Massachusetts (DDC Report AD 742259).

Klopf, A. H. (1975) A comparison of natural and artificial intelligence. *ACM Special Interest Group on Artificial Intelligence (SIGART) Newsletter,* No. 52 (June).

Koike, H., Kandel, E. R., and Schwartz, J. H. (1974) Synaptic release of radioactivity after intrasomatic injection of choline-$^3$H into an identified cholinergic interneuron in abdominal ganglion of Aplysia California. *J. Neurophysiol.* 37:815-827.

Konorski, J. (1948) *Conditioned reflexes and neuron organization.* Cambridge University Press, New York.

Konorski, J. (1950) Mechanisms of learning. *Symp. Soc. Exp. Biol.* 4:409-431.

Lighthill, J. (1973) Artificial intelligence: A general survey. *Artificial intelligence: A paper symposium.* Science Research Council Pamphlet, Science Research Council, State House, High Holburn, London.

Lorenz, K. (1970) On killing members of one's own species. *Bull. Atom. Sci.* 26(8):2-5.

Luria, A. R. (1978) The human brain and conscious activity. In *Consciousness and self-regulation: Advances in research and theory* Vol. 2 (eds. G. E. Schwartz and D. Shapiro), Plenum Press, New York, pp. 1-35.

MacLean, P. D. (1962) New findings relevant to the evolution of psychosexual functions of the brain. *J. Nerv. Ment. Dis.* 135:289-301.

MacLean, P. D. (1964) Man and his animal brains. *Mod. Med.* 32:95-106.

Marr, D. (1969) A theory of cerebellar cortex. *J. Physiol.* 202:437-470.

McCulloch, W. S., and Pitts, W. (1943) A logical calculus of the ideas immanent in nervous activity. *Bull. Math. Biophys.* 5:115-137. (Reprinted in McCulloch, W. S. (1965) *Embodiments of mind.* M.I.T. Press, Cambridge, Mass., pp. 19-39.)

McIntyre, A. K. (1953) Synaptic function and learning. *Abstracts of 19th International Physiological Congress,* pp. 107-114.

Meldrum, B. S. (1966) Electrical signals in the brain and the cellular mechanisms of learning. *Aspects of learning and memory* (ed. D. Richter). Basic Books, New York, pp. 100-120.

Melzack, M., and Wall, P. D. (1965) Pain mechanisms: A new theory, *Science* 150:971-979.

Miller, N. E. (1957) Experiments on motivation *Science* 126:1271.

Milner, P. M. (1957) The cell assembly: Mark II, *Psychol. Rev.* 64(4): 242-252.

Minsky, M. (1954) *Neural nets and the brain-model problem.* Ph.D. dissertation, Princeton University, Princeton, New Jersey (available from University Microfilms, Ann Arbor, Michigan.)

Minsky, M. (1969a) Matter, mind and models. In *Semantic information processing* (ed. Marvin Minsky). M.I.T. Press, Cambridge, Mass., pp. 425–432.

Minsky, M. (1969b) *Semantic information processing.* M.I.T. Press, Cambridge, Mass.

Minsky, M. (1975) A framework for representing knowledge. In *The psychology of computer vision* (ed. P. H. Winston). McGraw-Hill, New York, pp. 211–277.

Minsky, M., and Papert, S. (1969) *Perceptrons: An introduction to computational geometry.* M.I.T. Press, Cambridge, Mass.

Minsky, M., and Papert, S. (1977) Artificial intelligence from the perspective of neurodevelopmental epistemology. *Brain Theory Newsletter* 3:11–15.

Morrell, F. (1961) Effect of anodal polarization on the firing pattern of single cortical cells. *Ann. New York Acad. Sci.* 92:860–876.

Morrell, F., and Baker, L. (1961) Effects of drugs on secondary epileptogenic lesions. *Neurology* 11:651.

Morrell, F., Proctor, F., and Prince, D. A. (1965) Epileptogenic properties of subcortical freezing. *Neurology* 15:744.

Morrell, F. (1969) Physiology and histochemistry of the mirror focus. In *Basic mechanisms of the epilepsies* (eds. H. H. Jasper, A. A. Ward, Jr., and A. Pope). Little, Brown and Company, Boston, pp. 357–374.

Moruzzi, G., and Magoun, H. W. (1949) Brain stem reticular formation and activation of the EEG. *Electroencephalogr. Clin. Neurophysiol.* 1: 455–473.

Nathan, P. W. (1976) The gate-control theory of pain: A critical review, *Brain* 99:123–158.

Nauta, W. J. H. (1960) Some neural pathways related to the limbic system. In *Electrical studies on the unanesthetized brain* (eds. E. R. Rainey and D. S. O'Doherty). Hoeber, New York, pp. 1–16.

Newell, A. (1970) Remarks on the relationship between artificial intelligence and cognitive psychology. In *Theoretical approaches to nonnumerical problem solving* (eds. R. B. Banerji and M. D. Mesarovic). Springer-Verlag, Berlin.

Newell, A., Shaw, J. C., and Simon, H. (1957) Empirical explorations with the logic theory machine. *Proceedings of the Western Joint Computer Conference* 15:218–239. (Reprinted in Feigenbaum, E. A., and Feldman, J. (1963) *Computers and thought.* McGraw-Hill, New York, pp. 109–133.)

Newell, A., Shaw, J. C., and Simon, H. (1958) Chess playing programs and the problem of complexity. *IBM J. Res. Dev.* 2:320–335. (Reprinted in Feigenbaum, E. A., and Feldman, J. (1963), *Computers and thought*, McGraw-Hill, New York, pp. 39–70.)

Nilsson, N. J. (1965) *Learning machines.* McGraw-Hill, New York.

Nilsson, N. J. (1974) *Artificial intelligence.* Artificial Intelligence Center Technical Note 89, Stanford Research Institute, Menlo Park, California; also presented at IFIP Congress 74, Stockholm, Sweden, August 5-10, 1974.

Olds, J. (1962) Hypothalamic substrates of reward. *Physiol. Rev.* 42:554.

Olds, J. (1975) Mapping the mind onto the brain. In *The neurosciences: Paths of discovery* (eds. F. G. Wordon, J. P. Swazey, and G. Adelman). M.I.T. Press, Cambridge, Mass., pp. 374-400.

Olds, J. (1976) Brain stimulation and the motivation of behavior. In *Progress in Brain Research* Vol. 45 (eds. M. A. Corner and D. F. Swaab). Elsevier North-Holland, New York, p. 414.

Olds, J., and Milner, P. (1954) Positive reinforcement produced by electrical stimulation of septal area and other regions of rat brain. *J. Comp. Physiol. Psychol.* 47:419-427.

Palmieri, G., and Sanna, R. (1960) *Methodos* 12 (48).

Pavlov, I. P. (1927) *Conditioned reflexes.* Oxford University Press, New York.

Penfield, W. (1969) Epilepsy, neurophysiology, and some brain mechanisms related to consciousness. *Basic mechanisms of the epilepsies* (ed. H. H. Jasper, A. A. Ward, Jr., and A. Pope). Little, Brown and Company, Boston, pp. 791-805.

Penfield, W. (1975) *The mystery of the mind.* Princeton University Press, Princeton, New Jersey.

Pepper, S. C. (1960) A neural-identity theory of mind. In *Dimensions of mind* (ed. S. Hook). Collier Books, New York, pp. 45-61.

Poschel, B. P. H., and Ninteman, F. W. (1963) *Life Sci.* 3:782.

Powers, W. T. (1973) *Behavior: The control of perception.* Aldine Publishing Company, Chicago.

Pratt, J. B. (1937) *Personal realism.* MacMillan, New York.

Pribram, K. H. (1966) Some dimensions of remembering: Steps toward a neuropsychological model of memory. In *Macromolecules and behavior* (ed. J. Gaito). Academic Press, New York, pp. 165-187.

Pribram, K. H. (1971) *Languages of the brain.* Prentice-Hall, Englewood Cliffs, New Jersey.

Pribram, K. H. (1976) Executive functions of the frontal lobes. In *Mechanisms in transmission of signals for conscious behavior* (ed. T. Desiraju). Elsevier, New York, pp. 303-322.

Proctor, F., Prince, D., and Morrell, F. (1966) Primary and secondary spike foci following depth lesions. *Arch. Neurol.* 15:151.

Puccetti, R. (1973) Brain bisection and personal identity. *Brit. J. Phil. Sci.* 24:339-355.

Ramon y Cajal, S. (1911) *Histologie du systeme nerveux de l'homme et des vertebres,* Vol. 2. Maloine, Paris.

Rashevsky, N. (1938) *Mathematical biophysics.* University of Chicago Press, Chicago, Illinois.

Rescorla, R. A., Wagner, A. R., (1972) A theory of Pavlovian conditioning: Variations in the effectiveness of reinforcement and non-reinforcement. In *Classical conditioning II: Current research and theory* (eds. A. H. Black and W. F. Prokasy). Appleton-Century-Crofts, New York.

Rimland, B. (1964) *Infantile autism: The syndrome and its implications for a neural theory of behavior.* Prentice-Hall, Englewood Cliffs, New Jersey.

Rochester, N., Holland, J., Haibt, L. H., and Duda, W. L. (1956) Tests on a cell assembly theory of the action of the brain. *IRE Trans. Inf. Theory* IT-2:80-93.

Roffwarg, H. P., Muzio, J. N., and Dement, W. C. (1966) Ontogenetic development of the human sleep-dream cycle. *Science* 152:604.

Rosenblatt, F. (1957) *The perceptron: A perceiving and recognizing automaton, project PARA.* Cornell Aeronautical Laboratory Report 85-460-1, Buffalo, New York.

Rosenblatt, F. (1960) *On the convergence of reinforcement procedures in simple perceptrons.* Cornell Aeronautical Laboratory Report VG-1196-G-4, Buffalo, New York.

Rosenblatt, F. (1962) *Principles of neurodynamics.* Spartan Books, New York.

Roszak, T. (1972) *Where the wasteland ends: Politics and transcendence in post-industrial society.* Doubleday, New York.

Routtenberg, A. (1978) The reward system of the brain. *Sci. Am.* 239 (5): 154-164.

Rowland, V., and Goldstone, M. (1963) *Electroenceph. Clin. Neurophysiol.* 15:474.

Rusinov, V. S. (1953) An Electrophysiological analysis of the connecting function in the cerebral cortex in the presence of a dominant area, *Abstract of the Nineteenth International Physiological Conference,* pp. 719-720.

Russell, B. (1921) *The analysis of mind.* MacMillan, New York.

Russell, I. S. (1966) Animal learning and memory. In *Aspects of learning and memory* (ed. D. Richter). Basic Books, New York, pp. 121-171.

Sakai, M., Swartz, B. E., Woody, C. D. (1979) Controlled microrelease of pharmacologic agents: Measurements of volume ejected *in vitro* through fine tipped glass microelectrodes by pressure. *Neuropharmacology* 18:209-213.

Sampson, J. R. (1969) *A neural subassembly model of human learning and memory.* Technical Report, Computer and Communication Sciences Department, The University of Michigan, Ann Arbor.

Samuel, A. L. (1959) Some studies in machine learning using the game of checkers. *IBM J. Res. Dev.* 3:211-229. (Reprinted in Feigenbaum, E. A., and Feldman, J. (1963) *Computers and thought,* McGraw-Hill, New York, pp. 71-105.)

Segundo, J. P., Takenaka, T., and Encabo, H. (1967) Electrophysiology of bulbar reticular neurons. *J. Neurophysiol* 30:1194-1220.

Selfridge, O. G. (1959) Pandemonium: A paradigm for learning, *Proceedings of Symposium on Mechanisation of Thought Processes,* Natl. Phys. Lab., Teddington, England. Her Majesty's Stationery Office, London, 2 vols., pp. 511-529.

Sem-Jacobsen, C. W., and Torkildsen, A. (1960) Depth recording and electrical stimulation in the human brain. *Electrical studies on the unanesthetized brain* (eds. E. R. Ramey and D. S. O'Doherty). Harper, New York.

Sharpless, S. K. (1964) Reorganization of function in the nervous system-use and disuse. *Ann. Rev. Physiol.* 26:357-388.

Sherrington, C. S. (1941) *Man on his nature.* MacMillan, New York.

Skinner, B. F. (1938) *The behavior of organisms: An experimental analysis.* Appleton-Century, New York.

Skinner, B. F. (1971) *Beyond freedom and dignity.* Knopf, New York.

Smith, B. H. and Kreutzberg, G. W. (1976) Neuron-target cell interactions, *Neurosci. Res. Prog. Bull.* 14 (3):217-453.

Sommerhoff, G. (1974) *Logic of the living brain.* Wiley, New York.

Spencer, W. A., Thompson, R. F., and Neilson, D. R., Jr. (1966a) Alterations in responsiveness of ascending and reflex pathways activated by iterated cutaneous afferent volleys. *J. Neurophysiol.* 29:240-252.

Spencer, W. A., Thompson, R. F., and Neilson, D. R., Jr. (1966b) Decrement of ventral root electrotonus and intracellulary recorded PSP's produced by iterated cutaneous afferent volleys. *J. Neurophysiol.* 29:253-273.

Sperry, R. W. (1966) Brain bisection and consciousness. *Brain and conscious experience* (ed. J. C. Eccles). Springer-Verlag, New York, pp. 298-308.

Sperry, R. W. (1975) In search of psyche. In *The neurosciences: Paths of discovery* (eds. F. G. Worden, J. P. Swazey, and G. Adelman). M.I.T. Press, Cambridge, Mass., p. 429.

Spinelli, D.. N. (1970) OCCAM: A computer model for a content addressable memory in the central nervous system. In *Biology of memory* (eds. K. Pribram and D. Broadbent). Academic Press, New York, pp. 293-306.

Spinelli, D. N., and Jensen, F. E. (1979) Plasticity: The mirror of experience. *Science* 203:75-78.

Stein, L. (1964a) Reciprocal action of reward and punishment mechanisms. In *The role of pleasure in behavior* (ed. R. G. Heath). Harper and Row, New York, pp. 113-139.

Stein, L. (1964b) Self-stimulation of the brain and the central stimulant action of amphetamine. *Fed. Proc.* 23:836.

Stein, L. (1967) Psychopharmacological substrates of mental depression. *Antidepressant drugs* (eds. S. Garattini and N. M. G. Dukes). Excerpta Medica Foundation, Amsterdam, pp. 130-140.

Stein, L. (1968) Chemistry of reward and punishment. *Psychopharmacology: A review of progress: 1957-1967* (ed. D. H. Efron). U.S. Government Printing Office, Washington, D.C., pp. 105-123.

Stein, L., and Seifter, J. (1961) Possible mode of antidepressive action of imipramine. *Science* 134:286.

Stein, L., and Wise, C. D. (1971) Possible etiology of schizophrenia: progressive damage to the noradrenergic reward system by 6-hydroxydopamine. *Science* 171:1032.

Sutton, R. S. (1978a) *A unified theory of expectation in classical and instrumental conditioning.* Unpublished undergraduate thesis, Stanford University.

Sutton, R. S. (1978b) Single channel theory: A neuronal theory of learning. *Brain Theory Newsletter* 3 (3-/-4):72-75.

Sutton, R. S., Barto, A. G. (1979) *Toward a modern theory of adaptive networks I: Expectation and prediction.* COINS Technical Report 79-17, Computer and Information Science Department, University of Massachusetts, Amherst.

Tanzi, E. (1893) I fatti e la induzione nell' odierne istologia del sistema nervoso. *Riv. sper. Freniat.* 19:149.

Teitelbaum, P., and Epstein, A. N. (1962) *Psychol. Rev.* 69:74.

Thatcher, R. W., John, E. R. (1977) *Foundations of cognitive processes: Functional neuroscience* (Vol. 1). Lawrence Erlbaum Associates, Hillsdale, New Jersey.

Thomas, L. (1974) *The lives of a cell.* Viking Press, New York.

Thompson, R. F., and Spencer, W. A. (1966) Habituation: A model phenomenon for the study of neuronal substrates of behavior. *Psychol. Rev.* 73:16-43.

Thorpe, W. H. (1956) *Learning and instinct in animals.* Methuen, London.

Tonnies, J. F. (1949) Die erregungssteuerung im zentralnervensystem, *Arch. Psychiat. Nervenkr.* 182:478-535.

Uttal, W. R. (1978) *The psychology of mind.* Lawrence Erlbaum Associates, Hillsdale, New Jersey.

Uttley, A. M. (1966) The transmission of information and the effect of local feedback in theoretical and neural networks. *Brain Res.* 2:21-50.

Uttley, A. M. (1975) The informon in classical conditioning. *J. Theor. Biol.* 49:355-376.

Uttley, A. M. (1976a) A two-pathway informon theory of conditioning and adaptive pattern recognition. *Brain Res.* 102:23-35.

Uttley, A. M. (1976b) Simulation studies of learning in an informon network. *Brain Res.* 102:37–53.

Uttley, A. M. (1976c) Neurophysiological predictions of a two-pathway informon theory of neural conditioning. *Brain Res.* 102:55–70.

Wada, J. A., and Cornelius, L. R. (1960) Functional alteration of deep structures in cats with chronic focal cortical irritative lesions. *Arch. Neurol* 3:425.

Walter, W. G., Cooper, R., Aldridge, V. J., McCallum, W. C., and Winter, A. L. (1964) Contingent negative variation; an electric sign of sensori-motor association and expectancy in the human brain. *Nature* 203:380.

Ward, Jr., A. A., Jasper, H. H., and Pope, A. (1969) Clinical and experimental challenges of the epilepsies. *Basic mechanisms of the epilepsies* (eds. H. H. Jasper, A. A. Ward, Jr., and A. Pope). Little, Brown and Company, Boston, pp. 1–12.

Weil, J. L. (1974) *A neurophysiological model of emotional and intentional behavior*. Thomas, Springfield, Illinois.

Weizenbaum, J. (1972) On the impact of the computer on society. *Science* 176:609–614.

Weizenbaum, J. (1976) *Computer power and human reason*. Freeman, San Francisco.

Widrow, B., and Hoff, M. E. (1960) *Adaptive switching circuits*. Stanford Electronics Laboratories Technical Report 1553-1, Stanford University, Stanford, California.

Widrow, B. (1962) Generalization and information storage in networks of adaline neurons. In *Self-organizing systems–1962* (eds. M. C. Yovits, G. T. Jacobi, and G. D. Goldstein), Spartan Books, Washington, D.C., pp. 435–461.

Widrow, B., Groner, G. F., Hu, M. J. C., Smith, F. W., Specht, D. F., and Talbert, L. R. (1963) Practical applications for adaptive data-processing systems. *1963 WESCON Paper 11.4* (Pt. 7) 7.

Wiener, N. (1948) *Cybernetics.* Wiley, New York.

Wilkins, M. G. (1970) *Neural modelling: methodology, techniques and a multilinear model for information processing.* Biological Computer Laboratory Technical Report No. 19, University of Illinois, Urbana, Illinois (DDC Report AD 727770).

Wise, C. D., and Stein, L. (1969) Facilitation of brain self-stimulation by central administration of norepinephrine. *Science* 163:299.

Wise, C. D., and Stein, L. (1970) Amphetamine: Facilitation of behavior by augmented release of norepinephrine from the medial forebrain bundle. *Amphetamines and related compounds* (eds. E. Costa and S. Garanttini). Raven, New York, pp. 463–485.

Woody, C. D. (1974) Mechanisms underlying blink conditioning in the cat. *Cellular mechanisms subserving changes in neuronal activity* (eds. C. D. Woody, et al.). Brain Information Service, University of California, Los Angeles, pp. 5-12.

Woody, C. D. (1977) Changes in activity and excitability of cortical auditory receptive units of the cat as a function of different behavioral states. *Ann. New York Acad. Sci.* 290:180-199.

Young, J. Z. (1951) Growth and plasticity in the nervous system. *Proc. Roy. Soc.* B 139:18-37.

Young, J. Z. (1966) *The memory system of the brain.* University of California Press, Berkeley.

# author index

# subject index